Alive with Vigor

Alive with Vigor

Robert Earl Sutter III

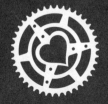

Alive with Vigor

Robert Earl Sutter III

ISBN 9781934620472

First Published February 15, 2014

Microcosm Publishing
636 SE 11th Ave
Portland, OR 97214

Designed and Edited by Joe Biel
Line Edited by Lauren Hage

Distributed by IPG

TABLE OF CONTENTS

Introduction
Robert Earl Sutter III

Everything we do and don't do contributes to our health and to the health of everyone around us. We're all interconnected in a way that sometimes seems terribly complicated, but sometimes incredibly simple: if we go on a drinking binge for three days, wreck our immune system, and catch the flu, we should not be surprised. Note to self: take it easy!

What is healthy for one person may not be healthy for another. Priorities can be different with our different bodies and you may find contradictions in this book! We are not pretending to know what is best for everyone, only to share our experiences. Sometimes you need to hear others' stories to realize what is going on with yourself. Reading these accounts can be helpful as you reflect on your own.

Not everyone has the same access to health care, money, a supportive network of friends and family, and privilege. Some of this advice might not be appropriate or possible for you, but the stories can inspire your own self-care, community care, and spark conversations with others about ways to be healthy.

The recent death of Elyse Mary Stern, someone close in our community here in Minneapolis, while riding her bicycle has made me reconsider the delicate hold on life that we have. I considered my own behavior, like cycling on our city streets, and made a choice to be more cautious and aware. I looked at my clunker of a bike: bad brakes, skipping drive train, no lights. I counted my money. What good would that money do if I was killed because my bicycle failed at a crucial moment? I broke open the piggy bank and got a decent ride: two working brakes, a good drive train, perfect wheels, and a front and back light for night riding. I'm cautious at every intersection and attempt to be mindful all the time while riding. When riding a bike or driving a car, it is essential to our survival to pay great attention to what we are doing when we are doing it. If you're out drinking and somebody offers you a chance to sleep it off before going home, please take the offer. No drunk driving.

Sometimes the thing to consider is how our injury, harm, or death would affect those close to us, even if we are terribly depressed or having a hard time and ceasing to care. Sometimes rebuilding your close relationships and having a heart-to-heart about your problems can provide those reasons to live that were escaping you or had gone forgotten. Sometimes seeing how much you mean to other people happens because of a trauma, tragedy, or a diagnosis and it can bring your community closer together.

Everyone in this book is a survivor of their experiences and there is much to learn. I hope this book will inspire conversations about health so we can continue learning from each other, and to live with vigor!

DEALING WITH EMOTIONS
Will Meek PhD

When I was a younger dude, there were only two emotions I could deal with, joy and anger. Any other feelings I had about myself, my relationships, or the world around me either became those two, or left me a confused and miserable mess. Any type of emotional pain was overwhelming, and by the time I was 17, I made a deal with myself to eliminate all emotions from my life. By focusing on logic and reason at all times, I could avoid the rollercoaster of emotions that I was prone to.

After a few months I actually got pretty good at this. I could carefully analyze any situation that generated the slightest bit of feeling, and maintained a reasonable equilibrium most of the time. Unfortunately, there was a dark side. I started to become detached from the most important people in my life, and generally started to lose motivation for things I previously loved.

What I did was find a way to circumvent something that makes us all human. Emotions are signals about what is happening in our lives, and they also help us form healthy attachments, stay motivated, plan for the future, show that we are hurting, and avoid danger. Eliminating that stuff made my life feel flat and meaningless.

A few years later I made some radical changes to embrace my feelings, and figure out how to ride their occasionally terrifying waves, and corral their power when I needed to stay in control. I also became a psychologist that focuses on emotions, and have been working to help other people manage their feelings better than I did.

If you are someone who has some issues dealing with your feelings, whether they be anger, anxiety, depression, grief, excitement, lust, or anything else, there are a few things you should know. These five steps are based on brain research and backed up by real life experience, and they were key for me learning to deal with my feelings too. To make the most of this, next time you are having a strong emotion, go through each step in order, which should help you have a deeper understanding of what is happening, and what to do next.

1. Sensing

The building blocks of emotions are in the physical sensations and automatic impulses we experience. So the first step in dealing with your emotions is to scan your body and specifically identify the types of sensations and motivations you are having. Is your stomach turning? Is your jaw clenched? Is there a lump in your throat? Is your face flush? Do you want to throw something through a wall? One mistake people make is skipping over this step entirely, which leaves us out of tune with our body. Another is when we deny that the sensations exist, or assume them to be something other than part of an emotional experience, like saying "I'm just tired".

2. Naming

Once you have the feelings down, it is important to accurately name the emotion. The mistakes people make here are mislabeling it, or using generic words that do not get it exactly right. For example, using words like "weird," "upset," or "bothered" all have a variety of meanings. There is more power and ability to work with the emotion when using words like "anxious," "sad," or "angry" instead. Additionally, we often have blends of several emotions at a time, or conflicting emotions, which makes this part even more difficult. Having a good emotional vocabulary is an important part of this, so look below for a list of emotion words.

3. Attributing

After you have the right emotion, it is key to accurately determine what caused it. Sometimes this is obvious, whereas other times emotions seem to "come out of nowhere" or "for no reason." Emotions are almost always triggered by something, but the triggers may be unknown to us. A common explanation for emotions coming "out of nowhere" is that the emotion was present, but was only consciously experienced when there was space for it, like when doing a mindless task, or laying down at night to sleep. A mistake people make in this step is attributing the emotion exclusively to one thing. For example, say a person that just had an argument, and then became enraged in traffic. In this step, we'd say that the anger was immediately provoked by the traffic, but the strength of the emotion is likely due to the earlier argument.

4. Evaluating

In this step we ask ourselves how we feel about having the emotion. We all have different answers to this based on our identity, culture, and comfort with certain emotions. For example, someone may feel perfectly comfortable being angry, but feel very uncomfortable feeling sad. I often hear people say things like "I'm angry that I'm angry." Unfortunately, this extra feeling means that the intensity of the emotional experience will increase because discomfort, shame, or something else has been added to sadness.

Things can get complicated here if we do not accept or value the emotions that we are experiencing. I generally promote the idea that all of our emotions are valid and have value, even if it is just a signal that something is happening within us, or in the world. Judgment can be reserved for our actions related to our emotions (step 5), but spare the emotions themselves, and instead work to accept that they are there and have a purpose.

5. Acting

After this is complete, we are left with choices about how to proceed. Sometimes when we have a flash of a very strong emotion, the action will just happen. But for emotions that linger or come and go in lower doses, we get to decide whether and how we will express it, and how to cope with it. The key here is that if we think ahead about what kind of action to take, we can avoid making mistakes in our lives based on sparked emotion. So developing a set of coping strategies and communication skills is also important for this step, and you can find some options elsewhere in this book.

List of Emotions

This is not an exhaustive list, but may be able to help you expand your emotion vocabulary.

Fear: anxious, avoidant, cautious, concerned, frozen, insecure, intimidated, guarded, overwhelmed, panicked, stressed, tense, terrified, trapped, vulnerable, worried.

Anger: aggressive, bitter, cold, competitive, defensive, disgusted, disrespected, enraged, frustrated, hostile, irritated, jealous, mad, outraged, resentful, revolted.

Sadness: apathetic, depressed, disheartened, disappointed, disillusioned, embarrassed, grief-stricken, guilty, hurt, lonely, needy, regretful, rejected, shameful, stuck, tired, weak.

Joy: blissful, brave, confident, connected, ecstatic, energized, excited, friendly, happy, hopeful, loved, loving, proud, powerful, rebellious, relieved, relaxed, spiritual, strong, thankful, touched, tough, warm

Self-Conscious Emotions: guilt, shame, embarrassment, and pride.

GROWING INTO SELF-CARE
James DeWitt

When I moved to Minneapolis I had some loose ideas about self-care and health. I had gone to a small liberal arts college and got exposed to a lot of people and projects that had a health focus, including the Icarus Project, and I was heading down a path of using less psych meds, using herbal medicine, "dealing with my shit," and eating differently than how I was raised. I thought I was pretty on top of things; I ate beets regularly, I tried out a yoga class, I came out as transgender and as a survivor of sexual abuse, I felt happier when I didn't have jobs, and I was forming an identity based in anarchy. I had a whole new skill set, right? I had a new vocabulary to work into my everyday framework: Accountability, community, white privilege, sex-positivity, anti-capitalism, anti-oppression. I was reading Crimethinc books and feeling like my life was changing and new things were possible.

Meanwhile, I was still using drugs and alcohol, still struggling with an eating disorder and other kinds of self-harm, and was barely starting to piece together the Big, Hard, Fucked Up things in my life. I could see the faintest image of how my experiences with manic depression, sexual abuse, self-harm, and anorexia were entwined in understanding my body, my gender, my sexuality, and my identity as queer. The totality of it all felt crushing, and drugs and alcohol were an acceptable way of coping in the scene I was a part of.

Before impulsively moving to Minneapolis, I had been living at home temporarily, working at a gas station where I ate my way through pop rocks-donuts-hot dogs-nachos-energy drinks all day long. In my first few days in Minneapolis, I polished off two or three jars of off-brand Jiffy peanut butter and several bags of apples. Without much money or a job or a place to live, I was mainly eating whatever anyone had dumpstered from Aldi. I got sick, and was throwing up pretty hard for a day or so.

I think of this as a turning point, an important moment in learning about self-care. The cause and effect of my food and environment had never been so clear to me before, as I had only ever eaten what was easily available around me. I experienced issues with internal bleeding and for the first time I was thoughtful and intentional about what I put into my body. Being so sick and miserable, I felt a strong desire to be somewhere quiet and safe, to sleep and heal and take care of myself—not the crowded, dirty house I was staying at. All of this led me to find more stable housing and think about the consequences of what I put into my body. A stable, quiet place allowed the loud, scary background noise from the trauma inside me to have somewhere to rest.

Since that moment, I've gotten connected to resources that have helped me deal with my past and taught me what self-care could look like. I found a new house to stay in, and was living with other queer people for the first time. I saw a whole new range of expression and identities claimed, different ways of forming relationships, exciting political and personal projects, and a space in my heart big enough to hold all of the complexity that used to feel so crushing.

I became interested in integrative medicine practices through friends, and the woo-ey environment I discovered in South Minneapolis. This felt like another turning point for me, to discover kinds of medicine that could deal with intangible issues like mental health and madness, trauma, and the disconnect I was feeling from my body. Through queer and trans youth organizations, I was connected with health practitioners and was encouraged to apply for state health insurance. Within a few months, I was receiving mental health counseling, found groups and orgs advocating for survivors of sexual abuse, and began receiving nutrition counseling, chiropractic care, cranial sacral massage, and acupuncture—all for cheap or free, just based on networking and finding people in my community. My therapist wrote me a letter to receive hormones. I was shocked at how quickly I could draw these resources together, and share them with my friends, co-workers, lovers, and roommates.

The more I get into self-care and healing, the more I find that other people in my life have similar struggles and a similar desire to figure it out. Many of my friends and lovers have dealt with what I am dealing with. Sometimes this feels hard, but other times it feels special to hold all of that together and support each other's needs. It seems like everyone has some good tip for how they deal with winter blues, migraines, insomnia, loneliness, hard times with family, and so on. It helps me to feel less alone, and I learn a lot from seeing how other people deal and cope as well as sharing what I know.

When I do my best self-care, it looks like this: I keep lots of good food at my house, and try not to eat gluten or soy because they are my migraine triggers, hurt my tummy, and make me even more spacey and weird than I usually am. I ride my bike, go on nice walks, run around with the kids I nanny for, and try to get exercise in a way that feels fun without being competitive or obsessive. It can be annoying when people say, "you should get some exercise," but it does help with my mental health. The problem is, when you are deeply depressed, how are you supposed to find the energy to go out and exercise? It works better when I can trick myself into doing active things instead of hyping myself up on a workout routine. When I can, I go to yoga, because it's a challenge to try and relax and be mindful of my body in that way. Supplements and herbs help my mental stability—especially 5-HTP, a natural serotonin booster! It's made a big difference for me. I try to keep little lists to remember what can help when I'm anxious, manic, having flashbacks, low self-esteem, stuck in my head, etc. Reaching out isn't always possible, and I'm working to find less harmful ways of dealing with what's in my head.

I learned some of the best skills through Dialectical Behavioral Therapy, which teaches funny acronym tips to learn emotional regulation, distress tolerance, interpersonal effectiveness, and mindful awareness. For example, one of my favorite acronyms is F.A.S.T., which stands for (be) Fair, (no) Apologies, Stick to your values, (be) Truthful. One of my favorite things about DBT is how far-fetched some of the acronyms are, but they really are effective. This is an interpersonal effectiveness skill, and has some strong associations with the non-violent communication model. Both promote being aware of your needs and advocating for them while being honest with yourself and others.

My most important skill is to keep up some psychic barriers between myself and my environment. What I've learned about energy/ the intangible/collective experiences is that there are ways to be open and vulnerable without being defenseless, and it's easy to get swept away in someone else's feelings and struggles, getting deep without losing yourself.

I learned this trick, called the Emotional Freedom Technique. It's a series of tapping on meridians in your body while saying these affirmations to yourself—and it's easy to find instructions online! You can do it practically anywhere, and it's helpful when I feel extra vulnerable. I also like "The Daily Energy Routine" from InnerSource. We hung it in our bathroom and my roommates and I would do it together as much as we could. It feels energizing and calming.

I'm trying to get real with those around me and build friendships that can support healing, growth, and being better friends—taking on less stuff and taking care of ourselves more. I'm sick of feeling loaded down, without the time to connect with the people I'm close to. Maybe this is where I'm going—figuring out how self-care makes me more capable of caring for others. I want more good walks and time together sober, wilding out without checking out or getting dangerous. I want to be extravagant to excess in the fancy food I can get for myself and my friends, and let our indulgence mean loving each other harder and treating ourselves to an even better quality of life; finding small magic in others and myself.

ANXIETY
Maddy Court

"Everyone gets anxious sometimes," is something I hear a lot. If living with generalized anxiety disorder for the past decade has taught me anything, it's that being open about your mental illness makes you a lint roller for unsolicited advice. Friends and medical professionals alike will tell you to resolve your crippling feelings of panic with activities out of a Pier 1 catalog e.g. rearrange the furniture in your room, make a collage from old magazines, light some candles. I was once administered lavender drops during a panic attack at an overnight school trip. I thought I was dying, but my breath smelled nice. In middle school, when my anxiety was at its peak, I was told to take a bubble bath on a weekly basis. So I could be anxious *and* wet, I guess.

I think one of the reasons people rarely understand the second half of the term "mental illness" is that like depression, the word anxiety is also used to describe healthy human reactions to difficult situations. To some people, mental illness is just another word for weakness or immaturity. The truth is that some brains just amplify feelings of stress and discomfort. Anxiety *hurts* and when you are hurting, no one ever has a right to negate or question your experiences.

I've been dealing with anxiety since the 5th grade. I'd spend hours worrying about what my body and face looked like, why my teachers didn't seem to like me as much as other students, whether or not my door-dashing dog would get hit by a speeding car, and the state of my parents marriage—basically, my thoughts were fixated on anything and everything that was out of my control. I'd worry until my stomach cramped up and my shoulders tensed up to my ears. Most nights, I'd sleep for an hour or two before waking up from heart palpitations. The worst thing about the physical affects of anxiety is that they feed the anxiety that caused them in the first place. When you can't sleep or eat, you become less and less mentally sound. Most people don't realize that mental illness can manifest itself physically.

My anxiety management CV isn't too impressive. The only professional therapy I've gotten was through my college's free counseling center. There was play-dough and classical music in the waiting room, so you can imagine how helpful my sessions were. But I will say this for myself: Over the past three years, I've gone from feeling intense anxiety almost every day to only once a month or so. Here's what I've found helps me and maybe you'll find it useful too:

1. One of the worst parts of feeling anxious is, at least to me, feeling irrational and powerless because I don't always know what's triggering my feelings. I like to visualize my anxiety as black tapioca balls in a glass of bubble tea. If I don't get rid of the gross tapioca balls, the bubble tea will overflow. My objective, then, is to scoop out the tapioca by removing myself from stressful situations, taking an Advil PM to fall sleep, eating an ultra-healthy meal, taking a yoga class, finding a dog to play with, and other acts of self-care. If you don't relate to the visual, make up your own.

2. Exercise. Even if it's just stretching in your room or walking around, you need the endorphins. It's also too easy to feel overwhelmed and powerless in bed.

3. I know it's not always possible, but you should never feel guilty about taking a personal day from school or work to recoup. On the other hand, sometimes it helps me to leave my room and be social. If I'm too anxious to engage with people, I'll see a movie or take a walk in a busy neighborhood alone. Hanging out alone used to make me self-conscious and antsy, but I promise that no one will even notice except you. New scenery and people can get you out of your head.

4. When my counselor suggested anti-depressants during my second year of college, I thought taking a pill would mean I was weak. Most of all, I was terrified of admitting that there was something abnormal about me. My counselor explained it as treating anxiety's root cause. Anxiety is often a manifestation or overlaying symptom of depression, so anti-depressants are often prescribed to treat anxiety. It can be better than letting it all boil over in a panic attack. I took Paxil, a pill that gives your brain a boost of synthetic serotonin, for a year and a half. It erased the highs and lows of my emotional spectrum (I know everyone says that about psych meds, but that's exactly what Paxil did to me). I quit as soon as possible, but anti-depressants enabled me to function in school and work until I was in a better state to manage my anxiety. There's oodles of stigma around anti-depressants, but that's not a reason to discount them if you think they might help.

5. Alcohol is the worst thing for your anxious-ass. Stay away from it. Weed makes me feel paranoid and jumpy but tons of responsible, functional adults find it helpful. It's probably safe to say that it's less harmful than pharmaceuticals.

Anxiety isn't who I am and it's not who you are, either. I hear people say things like, "you are not your mental illness" or "you are more than what you are going through." And it's true! Nevertheless, anxiety taught me to be emphatic and aware of the privileges afforded by mental health. Everyone is equipped to handle challenges differently. To cope with anxiety is to fight for my boundaries, my right to care for myself, and my right to exit unhealthy situations. I want to honor these lessons because when it's possible to do more than just survive a rough situation, it can feel pretty kickass.

MARATHON RUNNING IS PUNK!

Andre Hewitt O'Donnell

I used to *hate* running. Without fail, I was *always* the last kid during gym class runs and the multitude of soccer teams my parents forced me to join. Combined with being fat and having a penchant for general rebellion (read: punk rock politics, attempts at pseudo vegetarianism, listening to The Smiths, etc.), *running and I did not mix.* I associated running with exercise; exercise with group sports; group sports with the popular, preppy kids who had an interest in making fun of me. In high school, I joined marching band as a way to *avoid* taking gym class.

Sadly, not a single adult ever told my Young Self that fitness did not have to be *forced* group sports teams, gym classes, and weight loss summer camps. No adult ever said, "Hey Andre, health and fitness comes in all body shapes and sizes!" My mentors, idols, and self-projected role models were alcoholic band teachers and moody pop singers (read: Morrissey). There were no voluptuous punk rock yoga teachers, no heavily-tattooed ultra runners, and self-described anarchist activists lifting heavy weights. So for years, I continued to hate running, hate my body, and generally, pretty much hate myself.

I got sick of hating myself, so at some point I began the long, treacherous path towards self-love through years of psychotherapy, spirituality, relationships, traveling, and art. All this effort definitely helped but the path towards self-love took an unexpected twist during a routine physical. The physician informed me that I was pre-diabetic and most likely to get Type II Diabetes. Fortunately I had accrued enough self-esteem points to understand that the diet industry isn't punk either. When it got down to it, I realized that Hard Work is Punk. Years of making zines, dumpster diving food, scheming ways to live on the cheap, traveling, organizing events, and negotiating relationships in crowded punk houses was Hard Work too. It was an "aha!" light-bulb moment when I realized how punk-rock culture gave me the solid foundation I needed to become fit.

So I began this new chapter in my life with a Punk Ethic: Being Healthy Requires Hard Work. I know you don't want to hear those two words: *Hard Work.* But Hard Work is required for the satisfaction one gets from going on tour, recording an album, and making art. Relationships take Hard Work. Scouting your way through this world takes Hard Work. *There is nothing wrong with Hard Work.* If everything is handed down to you, do you appreciate what you have?

Or put it this way, chocolate chip cookies taste a lot better after a vigorous, stress relieving 8 mile run!

I began to get fit simply by eating real, healthy food (read: quinoa instead of 4 pieces of toast, blueberry smoothie instead of soda, dark chocolate instead of a candy bar) and working out. Initially, I joined a gym where I lifted weights and used the elliptical machine. Pushing aimlessly away on the elliptical machine for 45 minutes took a ton of mental fortitude. *It was not fun.* Eating whole, healthy food was probably the easiest part of my new Lifestyle Change. *Who doesn't like quinoa, apples, peanut butter, and blueberries?* I was bored with the fucking elliptical. This frustration led me to start running outside (because playing outside is fun!), starting with 1 mile, 2 miles, 3 miles, and onward. Each time I tacked an extra mile onto my run, my self-esteem rapidly increased. *Each new mile was like sticking the middle finger to all the kids in school who made fun of me for being weird, it was like saying "weird people can run, in fact they sometimes might run faster than you!"*

As the miles increased, I signed up for short-distance races and from there, my first half-marathon. This particular half-marathon was life changing, as I ran the first portion in the snow. "If I can run 13.1 miles in the snow," I told myself "then I can run a marathon." From there, I ran my first marathon, then my second, twenty-fifth and beyond. "If I can run a marathon," the self-talk continued, "what else can I do?"

Some of my running highlights include running a marathon in the snow, running a marathon a week for four weeks in a row, and completing several 50K ultra marathons on pristine mountain trails. Despite these accomplishments, it is my daily morning runs that remind me that I am capable of more than I think. *Punk said, "You don't need society's approval to make art, just do it yourself." Running now says, "You don't need to follow society's standards to be fit, just go outside and move."*

While long distance running may not be everybody's preference, I encourage you to take the following guidelines and apply them to other areas in your life where you can practice health and fitness, such as cycling, yoga, walking, and martial arts.

Running is Punk because…

·   The Do It Yourself Ethic: When you go out for a run, you are solely relying on yourself. No machines. No gimmicks. Nobody else is doing it for you.

·   The healthier and happier you are, the more you are able to create change by being a positive role model.

·   Diversity: All sorts of people run. Making new friends and joining running communities shows you that people with different beliefs can still practice do it yourself ethics.

·   Running outside in all weather conditions is badass! Running through humidity, rain, snow, and wind pushes you. By doing this, you send the message that you are not going to let the weather break you down.

·   Feeling like a kid: Running outside gives you the freedom to run through alleyways, blocked streets, jumping over construction signs, and logs. When traveling, going for a run lets you explore new places.

·   Running is free! There are hundreds, if not thousands of free group runs and races all around the world. *Going for a walk is free. Doing yoga is free. Moving your body is free!*

OK, SO I THINK THIS COULD REALLY APPLY TO PEOPLE OF ANY SIZE, BUT I'VE GOTTA SPEAK FROM EXPERIENCE HERE, & MINE IS AS A FAT LADY. I GREW UP ABSORBING NEGATIVE BODY MESSAGES FROM ALL SIDES, & HIT A LOW POINT IN MY TEENS, WHEN THAT MIXED WITH THE STRESS OF ADOLESCENCE ADDED UP TO SOME SERIOUSLY FUCKED UP EATING. I LOST A LOT OF WEIGHT & FOLKS TOLD ME I LOOKED GREAT, BUT I FELT LIKE CRAP. THE WEIGHT ONLY STAYED OFF FOR A COUPLE YEARS, & I GAINED IT ALL BACK & MORE WHEN I STARTED LIVING ON MY OWN & EATING WHAT-EVER THE HELL I WANTED - WITHOUT REALLY KNOWING HOW TO TAKE CARE OF MYSELF. I STILL FELT LIKE CRAP.

IT TOOK A FEW MORE YEARS & A LITTLE MORE LIFE EXPERIENCE FOR ME TO FIGURE OUT HOW TO LIVE HAPPILY & HEALTHILY IN MY BODY.

NOW, I'M NOWHERE NEAR PERFECT, BUT I'VE LEARNED A THING OR TWO & I'D LIKE TO TAKE THIS OPPORTUNITY TO SUBMIT TO YOU MY PERSONAL RECIPE FOR BEING A **HAPPY, HEALTHY** *fat person!*

♡FIRST, **EAT WELL!** THIS SURE AS HELL DOESN'T MEAN DIETING - DON'T GET ME WRONG! I JUST MEAN, STEER YOURSELF MOSTLY IN THE DIRECTION OF FRUIT, VEGGIES, & WHOLE GRAINS. IF YOU DO THIS, & SURE, INCLUDE A CUPCAKE OR TWO FOR GOOD MEASURE (IF YOU WANT!), YOU'LL BE PRIMED TO FEEL YOUR BEST, AT WHATEVER WEIGHT YOUR BODY FALLS TO.

♡SPEAKING OF WEIGHT- **GET RID OF YOUR SCALE!** YOUR WEIGHT TELLS YOU NOTHING MORE THAN HOW YOUR BODY INTERACTS WITH GRAVITY - NOT HOW STRONG, HEALTHY, OR HOT YOU ARE.

♡ IF YOU DON'T KNOW HOW TO COOK,
LEARN TO COOK! BEING ABLE TO FEED
YOURSELF (& OTHERS) WILL HELP YOU FEEL
EMPOWERED, NOT TO MENTION TEACHING YOU
LOTS ABOUT FOOD, SAVING YOU $, & GUARANTEEING
THAT YOU KNOW WHAT'S GOING INTO WHAT YOU'RE
EATING! LEARNING TO COOK HAS BEEN ONE OF THE MOST
IMPORTANT COMPONENTS IN MY PERSONAL HEALTH-&-
HAPPINESS PLAN - I RECOMMEND IT HIGHLY!

♡ FIND SOME SORT OF PHYSICAL
♡ ACTIVITY YOU LIKE & **GO DO IT!**
BIKING IS FUN, & SO ARE SWIMMING,
DANCING, ICE SKATING, YOGA...

♡ **WEAR WHATEVER THE HELL YOU WANT!** I FIND
NOW THAT I'M MORE CONFIDENT IN MY BODY I ACTUALLY
FEEL MORE COMFORTABLE WEARING SOMEWHAT
FITTED CLOTHES. SOME PEOPLE LIKE LOOSE & FLOWY,
SOME SUPER TIGHT & SHORT- WHATEVER! REMEMBER
THE MOST IMPORTANT THING IS FOR YOU TO FEEL
GOOD, & LOOK GOOD TO YOURSELF.
EXPERIMENT! GO FOR IT!

♡ FIND SOME RAD FATTY
WRITINGS & **GET READING.**
THERE ARE LOTS OF GOOD
BOOKS & ZINES (FAT! SO?
IS A CLASSIC), & A MILLION
BLOGS OUT THERE-
GO FIND
'EM!

I CAN'T COVER HALF OF WHAT
I WANT TO IN
THESE PAGES!
CHECK OUT
OTHER PEOPLE'S
WORK ON
FATNESS &
RACE, HEALTH,
QUEERNESS,
DISABILITY
...

♡ SEARCH OUT YOUR RAD FATTY **COMMUNITY**! IF YOU'RE LUCKY, YOU CAN FIND AWESOME & LIKE-MINDED FOLKS IN YOUR TOWN. WHETHER OR NOT YOU'RE PHYSICALLY SURROUNDED BY THESE PEOPLE, THE INTERNET IS ANOTHER GREAT WAY TO CONNECT.

curvy

FAT FRIENDS ♥

Chubby

♡ EMBRACE WHATEVER **TERMS** FEEL COMFORTABLE TO YOU! THICK, CURVY, CHUBBY, PLUS-SIZED, RUBENESQUE, THE LIST GOES ON. I LIKE **FAT**. I DIDN'T ALWAYS, BUT ONCE I GOT USED TO IT, I FELL IN LOVE. IT'S SIMPLE, IT'S DESCRIPTIVE, & IT'S MINE. AND YOURS TOO, IF YOU WANT IT! - - - - - - - - - -

NOW, I WON'T PRETEND THAT THESE TIPS WILL DISSOLVE ALL FEELINGS OF SHAME OR SELF-DOUBT, BUT I HOPE MY EXPERIENCES WILL AT LEAST PLANT A SEED YOU CAN COME BACK TO WHEN FEELING BUMMED ABOUT YOUR BODY IS THREATENING TO GET THE BETTER OF YOU.

IN FACT, THERE'S ONE MORE INGREDIENT IN THIS RECIPE: **DON'T BEAT YOURSELF UP**! DON'T BEAT YOURSELF UP OVER YOUR BODY, <u>OR</u> IF YOU OCCASIONALLY FEEL LESS-THAN-GREAT ABOUT IT. BE YOUR OWN BEST ALLY. REMEMBER ALL THE GREAT THINGS ABOUT LIVING IN YOUR BODY, TAKE GOOD CARE OF IT, & SHOW THIS WORLD WHO'S HOT, HEALTHY, & AMAZING!

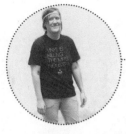

Back in the early stages of dating my now-husband, when we were only boyfriend and girlfriend, we had a conversation about some of the many traits we appreciated and admired in the other. Among them were the facts that we were both confident in ourselves, we didn't accept less than what we knew we deserved, and we communicated with such ease. While I didn't think much about it at the time, looking back on that conversation, I realize the positive signs that existed in our relationship from the beginning.

Of course, that doesn't mean that I have always had healthy relationships. In fact, like most adults, I have experienced my fair share of bad relationships, many of which could have been avoided if I had only paid attention to the red flags and trusted my gut instincts. But unfortunately, there is no comprehensive guide to how to succeed at love—and that's probably a good thing, as it's our experiences and mistakes that offer us the opportunity to learn and grow, and one-up ourselves in future relationships.

Still, while I am happy and satisfied with my love life, I did not come out of the dating world unscathed. It's inevitable that you will get hurt at some point—maybe even multiple times. You will also likely be the person hurting someone else at some point. And while it's enough heartbreak to make you question whether or not it's worth it, I can assure you that if you long for someone to love, the rollercoaster of emotions is completely worth it. Even so, I would like to offer a few pointers to guide you along the way.

The first thing to realize if you want to be successful at finding fulfilling partners is that you have to know yourself. Why? Well, if you aren't familiar with the ins and outs of yourself emotionally, intellectually, or physically, then how can you expect someone else to be? Maybe it sounds silly, since you would assume that of course you know yourself.

But this is a skill that not only includes knowing what you like or dislike or how you act in certain situations, but also understanding why. It involves becoming comfortable with who you are as a person, especially when you are alone. Pay careful attention to your moods and what makes you feel a certain way. Learn what makes you feel satisfied or accomplished with yourself. Find out how you reenergize, whether with others or while alone. Admit what your faults are and either change the ones that bother you or accept the ones that you think you can live with.

Only when this happens can you deeply comprehend and begin to appreciate yourself. And when you love yourself, your self-esteem skyrockets, and others begin to notice it too. Self-love is contagious—just think about how appealing confident people are. And when you emit an aura of self-satisfaction, people will wonder what is special about you and want to know you better. Most importantly, when you love yourself, you will want to preserve that state, and it can lead to better choices, where you seek out partners who also know and love themselves.

Another important tip for dating is to know what you want. While I am not the type of person who lives with regrets—an attitude that only stirs up feelings of self-loathing, which counteracts the self-love—I do often think about what drew me to certain individuals in life. Unfortunately, a lot of the people I dated were people I was with simply because I could be, and not because they were good for me, nor what I needed at the time. This is because before I really grew to love myself, I had relatively low standards, and that was reflected in those I dated and the way they made me feel.

It's often difficult to discover what we want or don't want in relationships without trial and error. Although relationships are often based on some kind of initial, mutual attraction, in part we also date people to discover how they fit with us. If we are lucky, we find mates who display the attributes we desire and want the same things we do. Sometimes, we also date people who are not on the same wavelength, but one or both parties aren't smart enough to realize it isn't working.

Then there are the relationships that I am all too familiar with, the ones where there is something wrong on multiple levels, but neither person does anything to change, fix, or end it. And what usually occurs is that one or both people are unhappy with the other, and unhappy with themselves. This is often because they overlook a fault or sacrifice a standard, and not just a minor one like how the other person is annoying when he or she eats, but a major one, like how your significant other makes you feel bad or ignores your feelings.

If my future self could talk to me in the past, I would tell her to stick to those standards. I don't know about you, but I spent a lot of time as a young girl and teenager making a list of personality traits that my "dream guy" had. Certainly, some of them were improbable, and others were plain corny, based on what I had seen in romantic happily-ever-after movies. But as I dated and made exceptions more, I became more and more disenchanted with this notion of romantic love, and it showed in who I opted to date. I dismissed my "standards" as unrealistic and instead settled for anyone who would show a bit of interest in me. I only wish I knew then how unhealthy and unsatisfiying this behavior would prove to be.

So make that list of what you want, regardless if it's a casual or serious relationship. For example, if you don't see the relationship as lasting but rather as a fun distraction, that's fine; you don't have to date someone who holds the same view as you about whether or not you wants kids if you don't plan to end up with him or her. But at the same time, if someone makes fun of you, makes you feel bad for a certain habit you have, or disrespects you, know where to draw the line. Sacrificing your own integrity to feel loved by someone who treats you like crap is not worth it, and chances are, if you stand up for yourself, you will feel empowered by your decision—something that holds far more social clout than having a boyfriend or girlfriend who makes you feel bad.

Finally, something I have found to be essential in my relationships is communication. In fact, I would venture to say that there is a direct correlation between how much you communicate openly with your partner and how healthy and satisfied you are capable of being in a relationship. Looking back, the unhappiest relationships in my life were ones when the communication was fractured or missing.

Why is communication important? One, it helps establish your needs and desires, and allows you to find out the same from your partner. Two, it builds trust between the pair, because you know where you stand and vice versa. Three, it helps eliminate unrealistic expectations and disappointments because what you want and expect from each other is already clearly stated. Whether you are discussing plans with your partner, opening up about vulnerabilities, or sharing what you need to be sexually satisfied, communication clears up the channels, as it removes any chance of doubt or confusion.

And it doesn't just end there. You have to work at these things— knowing yourself, sticking to your standards, and communicating openly—continually, in order for your relationships with others, and more importantly, with yourself, to thrive.

ANKLE SPRAIN
Greg

Running through the woods at night in Memphis, Tennessee, I am trying to catch a train that was pulling out, heading south. The rucksack on my back is heavy, because the March night was warm. I had put my cold weather clothes that I'd been wearing in Chicago the night before inside the bag. I should have thrown some of them away.

As I ran, I tripped over some fallen logs. It was dark and I had no light. I stood up and kept running. Then I tripped again. This time I felt a burning encompass my entire leg as my ankle bent further than it should have.

I lay down, writhing in pain as I listened to the train pull away, picking up speed.

I had no cell phone, no light, no money, very little food.

After 20 minutes I stood up on my good leg and carefully limped and crawled out of the woods. I found an abandoned industrial yard full of various machine parts, old cars, and two empty tractor trailers. I entered one trailer through the loading dock and laid out my sleeping bag.

In the morning I saw my ankle was so swollen that I couldn't see my ankle bones.

I lay there most of the day, happy that the place I'd stumbled into at night was still unoccupied in the day time, although it was a Sunday.

It was a bad sprain or maybe a break but I was alive and had shelter. I kept the foot elevated and I gave myself acupuncture, because I had training.

I figured that I needed to rest for a week. I didn't know anybody in Memphis. Nobody knew I was there.

At dusk I hobbled out of the scrapyard to see I was in the far outskirts of a residential area. In the vicinity I found a Zion Evangelical Baptist Church. I walked over to the back. Hallellueah, they had a water tap!

Even better, they had just had a picnic/barbeque and there were six aluminum trays each half full of delicious Southern food—black-eyed peas, okra, corn, bisquits and ham hocks ripe for the picking. Wooo-Hooo!

I stayed there three more days. Meditating on my throbbing ankle elevated against the backdrop of the abandoned scrapyard and the Tennessee sky. I was amazed that nobody walked through there that whole time.

On the fourth day the church food was developing a strange smell and a certain slime. I had to cook it good and hot on my little sterno stove to prevent poisoning myself.

At dusk I wrapped up my ankle with extra socks to stabilize it. I limped through the same woods with a newly crafted cane. Arriving at the tracks, I waited. Soon, a train pulled out and I caught it on the fly. My ankle hurt but I hoped that I would have a good 24 hours rest on the way to New Orleans.

The next day at dusk I crossed Lake Pontchartrain flat on my back, happy. The following morning I hobbled into the 9th ward to become another injured person in the wake of the Hurricane.

If you have any kind of sprain—think RICE / RACE: Rest, Ice/Acupuncture, Compress, Elevate. I didn't have ice in Memphis but rest, compression and elevation worked wonders. Only use ice on the 1st day or not at all, not after the acute swelling goes down. Ice can cause a chronic injury.

Don't overuse your injured part. Take it easy.

Once the swelling is gone but you need to get stagnant blood out of the area, alternate hot and cold to move the blood. You can also use herbs like Arnica, Myrrh, Safflower etc.

The most important aspect of surviving a dangerous situation is psychological. How you react to and interpret the experience is more important than the experience itself. You create your reality in that sense.

Everyone has their own path. Each individual will react to a given situation differently. Find your path and follow what's best for you. That is most important. You can tell people not to freak out but it's possible that in their experiences have been so unpleasant and traumatic that they carry it into every new experience. Experiences can result in never feeling basic security and some people can't just tell themselves that everything is okay.

The important thing to remember is that each moment is new. It is only connected to the past through you. If you convince yourself that you can't do something, then you can't. We need to be able to constantly let go of our experiences in life. While this is easier said than done, what's the point of trying to hold on to something that is impossible to grasp?

When you are stuck somewhere with no one to help, you will find something inside you.

When I get sick or injured it is often because I don't know what I am doing. It's usually because I'm hurrying and not listening to my inner voice or because I'm listening too much to other people or trying to please them. Other people are essential to my health but also have the capacity to ruin it. It's up to me to prevent that.

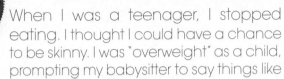

DOUBLE BODY IMAGE

Melanie Clothilde Double

When I was a teenager, I stopped eating. I thought I could have a chance to be skinny. I was "overweight" as a child, prompting my babysitter to say things like "you don't need that cookie." My mom would put me on her weird cabbage soup or slimfast shake diets. I was just a kid. Aside from being a naturally rounder human form, I gained weight as a child by turning to food to feel better when I was sad, which was often. But when I moved to live with my Mom across the country at age 13, I realized I could deal with the pain of existence in a new food related way. The feeling of hunger felt good. I liked walking through the day feeling dizzy and knowing it was making me skinnier. My anorexia was accompanied with self-mutilation, binge drinking, and anonymous sex.

It never got to the point where I had to be hospitalized. Some turning points happened within me. I started dating someone who respected me and was my equal in our weirdness. I knew I was queer, and I thankfully didn't have many problems with it, but my mom had taken my diary, where I had obsessively written about a girl I pined for. I found out she had taken it when one day I just couldn't find it. I didn't care but she later quasi-confessed, saying she read it, trying to suss out what drugs I was doing. Luckily, I was pretty open about my sexuality but my self-esteem, on the other hand, wasn't too shiny.

But dating a nice person that liked me caused me to revisit my self-esteem and make changes in my (non) eating: I became vegan. I don't remember what drew my interest to it. But I sent for a PETA kit and when it arrived, I looked at the pictures of the factory-farmed pigs and I just cried and cried for hours. Looking back, I wasn't just crying for the animals' pain. I started going to health food stores and experimenting with fake meats and soy shakes. I became excited about eating in a new way. Eating could have meaning for me, it was a political act. I felt a new sense of control in my life. I felt that I could mean something.

Things didn't happen instantaneously. I was still taking fen-phen pills occasionally. I moved to San Francisco, living in the tenderloin. I had no money for food. Not eating was different. I was going to City College, and would go into the Super Mercado, buy a 30 cent piece of bread and an apple for that day's meal. I still felt that dizzy feeling of "being skinny."

One day, I decided this was ridiculous. My fen-phen pills ran out, and I resolved to change my life so I could afford to eat properly. I didn't care how little money I had, somehow I would afford to eat. To this day, I make no qualms about buying myself whatever I want to eat, particularly healthy and wonderful things. I love to eat things that were grown nearby, without pesticides and nasty shit. This comes from a love for myself. My body is beautiful and unusual and I flaunt it so that others can be inspired to love their bodies. I now take care of myself emotionally as well as I can. I don't strive for any perfection, just equilibrium within myself.

I am endlessly inspired by the sexy fatties out there who know they are hot shit and flaunt it! Thank you.

CHANGE

Buck Angel

....

The hardest part of becoming me was being honest with myself. I had no idea what that meant, let alone that I could do it.

For years I struggled with self-loathing, insecurity, and hate. There was so much anger inside of me. "Why?" was always the question from everyone around me. My parents suffered along with me, and I am sure my sisters did as well.

It's not like I grew up in some horrible situation. I was raised in the San Fernando Valley in Southern California in a middle class neighborhood. It was all very "normal." Well, for a boy my youth was normal, but not for a girl who thought she was a boy. Or should I say I knew I was a boy. That was the problem.

Being a tomboy was okay and nobody questioned me when I was very young. My parents even called me Buck, from the time I was two or three years old, though my birth name was Susan.

But when I hit puberty and my body started to change, everyone started to question me, including my family. I began what would become a long history of self-mutilation and drug and alcohol abuse. Every day I would wake up thinking that I wanted to be a boy. Why did I have to be this other way? It was not common knowledge what a transsexual was in the 1970s. Gender was not considered something that you could choose.

Thankfully, in my youth I had sports. During high school I excelled in long-distance running. That gave me a sense of purpose like nothing else had before. In a way it saved my life, because I was so miserable. It's weird thinking about my tormented past because I am such a happy person now. I sometimes forget that right at this moment so many other people feel just the way I did. I'm hoping that by putting this out there you can believe that there is hope. Things can change; they sure did for me.

My grades in school were horrible and I had no focus. Running let me believe that I could be great at something. It always made me feel like a different person, and that was like magic. Eventually I became a star runner and won all kinds of competitions and awards and was sought after by many schools and organizations. But deep down I was still suffering because I was not dealing with my gender issues or my sexuality, so I got high and drunk.

That eventually was the downfall of my potentially great running career. Then it was just a matter of time before I became homeless and helpless. I truly felt that there was no way I could go on.

Somehow I had friends who still cared about me and literally picked me up off the street and took me to rehab. I got sober and have been now for over 20 years. But being high was always my security blanket and letting that go was so scary, but also powerful. The sobriety gave me a new clarity, a sort of vision that I could be the person I wanted to be—the man I wanted to become. Before getting my head clear from drugs and alcohol, I had not been able to see.

I did not know until then that I had the power to be myself, to say, "I don't care. I will be myself no matter what!"

You may not know you have the power. Nobody ever told me that I could be the person I wanted to be. They always said I was crazy because I dressed like a boy or that I was stupid because I was not doing well academically. What horrible things to say to a person.

Through sobriety I found my true self. If there is something you can take from my story it is to know that you can be whoever you want to be! Don't let people tell you otherwise. Do what your heart tells you is right. I did. It took me 28 years of denying myself before I finally got to be this person. And still, every day I am looking at the positives and changing for the better.

ADDICTION

David Chops

I started to party when I was 13 and it was super fun, and a way for me to check out, rebel, and be social. I was accepted by many of the party people and that feels awesome. So that's what I did for a long time. And yeah, I almost died a few times, but I didn't think much of it, and then I partied harder and more often. I felt crappy all the time, but I couldn't really remember what it felt like to be any other way.

At some point along the way I knew, somewhere deep inside, that this wasn't working anymore. But what else could I do? I tried to moderate. I tried hypnotherapy. I moved to a different town. Things got worse, and the feelings of desperation and guilt were overwhelming, I was so ashamed. I felt like nobody understood me. Had I always felt this way? My addiction consumed me in ways that I never knew possible.

For every addict I've met who has found a way to live without the use of drugs (alcohol is a drug), the story is always the same.

So when I was ready for a new way I asked for help.

It was a total surrender; I was losing this battle, and I was willing to admit I couldn't do this by myself. I was willing to do whatever it took. I asked a friend to drive me to a detox facility. I didn't have insurance and very little money, but they admitted me anyways.

When I was in the detox facility, some people visited who had been through what I was going through, and had come out of it and now had healthy, fulfilling lives without drugs. They learned from other addicts in recovery. I had heard of 12 step programs before and made fun of them with my friends. But nothing mattered more than not returning to the hell I was in, so I listened to what they had to say. I felt understood. They knew every little mind game I had been playing and how to get out of all the traps I had learned in order to keep using. They were in the process of recovery, and I wanted what they had so I did whatever they said to do. They told me to go to meetings. So I did.

I started going to N.A. (Narcotics Anonymous) and A.A. (Alcoholics Anonymous) meetings, two everyday. I liked the meetings in my area because the people were fun and stoked that I was there. Everyone was chill about mentioning the God/higher power dynamic often present in AA. If you're like me, having organized religion being shoved down your throat is enough to get in a fighting mood.

I learned how to not use anymore, how to live without using. If you suspect you have a problem, you probably do, and if you're like me, and you're not ready to stop using, you won't. That said, there were things I heard along the way that came in handy when I was ready.

Addiction is a progressive disease, it gets worse over time. Absolute abstinence of all mood and mind-altering substances is necessary for recovery. If there were a way to keep using, don't you think an addict would have figured it out by now?

Addicts who still use and people who are not addicts don't get it. Take the advice of those who have been through what you are going through and are now free from active addiction. Get away from the people and places that involve drug/alcohol use. Focus on new friends who don't use.

Give yourself a break, this is possibly the hardest, most fucked up, difficult, and confusing thing you will ever have to deal with. Allow yourself room to learn this new way of doing things. Practice meditation. This doesn't mean you have to buy a yoga mat and sit cross legged and burn incense. Don't be afraid to make it up as you go along. There is more than one right way to do this. Go for a walk or sit in a quiet place, or space out on a bus bench. This is part of giving yourself a break.

Don't use, no matter what.

It will get easier, with time. Do the work you need to in order to recover and the cravings will become less and less. It won't always be such a struggle to resist using.

Remember you are striving for progress, not perfection. Nobody gets it right all the time, so long as you're not using, you're doing pretty damn good!

Try new things out. I found that I didn't have to hide in the shadows anymore, there are so many places to explore.

It doesn't matter if you're shooting smack in your neck and sucking cock to pay for it, or you're a college kid hitting the bottle too hard. Everybody has a different rock bottom. If you're struggling with addiction you are worthy of recovery.

Get numbers of other addicts in recovery and give them a call if you are freaking out or just to see if you can actually call them. This will make their day and help them in their recovery as well.

Find the people who have some recovery time and listen to what they say, these will be the best teachers you can find. Go to 90 meetings in 90 days.

Understand that what you have been going through is really traumatic. It may take some time for you to realize just how hardcore what it is that you are doing, but you should know that you will have to heal emotionally, mentally, and physically. This takes time and work. You are fucked up and its gonna be a process to get through it.

Give it time. You are worthy of love. I doesn't matter what you've done in the past.

There is so much more. There is a whole world waiting for you. Some of it sucks, is hard, and feels bad. Some of it is exciting, is easy and feels good. and a million shades of grey in-between. Whatever happens in life, you never have to use again.

DEPRESSION

Alisha Yuen

Well, I don't know if I was ever all that social. I made friends with an outcast group at school because they saw I was always alone and took pity on me. There was Nguyen, a girl that was shipped over on a boat from Vietnam, probably the smartest of the bunch, Margarita, a Philipino girl, the fun beauty queen who had boyfriends well before we ever even considered it. Amber from Hawaii, fun and already engaged to a guy in Hawaii that was in the military. We had Robyn, half black and half white, her and Amber were two peas in a pod. Then we had Mary, an African American girl, who was the sweetest and close second to the smartest. Then me, the white girl, who was street smart and liked to drink and smoke weed before school, who cheated in math class and who loved heavy metal music.

That was middle school. The glory days. In the eighth grade my brother died and we moved to a rural area. No buses to catch to see the ocean or brother or friends to hang out with. So I would get loaded up on Co-Tylenols and go to high school, in a daze.

I hated everyone as they were so shallow though I met a girl, thank god, within my first two weeks. Gen, a tall, skinny, white girl. We met in math class when she asked, "Do you want to sit next to me?" She did most of the talking and I could tell this was a real human being, not superficial. She was caring and funny. She had a friend, Cheryl, who was the nut-case girl. She had a boyfriend involved with a gang and was of Mexican descent. There was never a dull moment with Cheryl. I remained in a cloud, a funk. After a year, Gen moved to Oregon. Cheryl and I "broke up" and I would spend most of my time by myself in the photo lab developing and manipulating photos. I tried to do well in school. At one point they even put me in honors classes. My counselor told me that I should attend college.

I did and I studied behavioral sciences and art and photography. Now majorly depressed. I had to have a stupid job to pay for my car to actually get to school and this sucked. Of course it was in retail where I had to be nice to strangers and ask them if they found everything alright. Had to actually force a smile and say fucking thank you, have a nice fucking day! I hated people. At school I did well, interested in what I was studying but I wouldn't talk to anyone. I hung out in my car and scribbled furiously in my notebook. I would write poetry, philosophies on life and stupid petty shit like how I'd like to kill myself.

Many times I thought of doing it. One night I drove to the ocean and walked into it clothes and all. I was a wuss. It was too cold. I tried strangling myself but that would never work. I can't tell you how many bags of apples I bought cause my biology teacher told us that if one would eat a hand full of apple seeds the cyanide could kill you. A long slow death.

Each time before I would attempt or even thought of killing myself. I would write a letter. It would take me a long time. I would usually sit in the bathtub and while writing, thinking of how cool it would be to slit my wrists. I would sob and write, eventually I was so worn out I'd go to bed. I thought to myself that I would take care of things the next day. Somehow I would awake refreshed and renewed.

I would carry out that day's events till it got so bad I'd do it again. I felt like I was under close scrupulation from the stupid, happy people that thought the world was alright. They were fine and living their lives and worried about petty things. Where had all the philosophers gone that actually cared about the human condition? Everyone was in oblivion, living thier perfect, glistening, shining happy lives, while the world was going to shit. Politically and socially fucked.

One morning, my mom took me out to breakfast. She started talking to me like a psychiatrist and said this was an intervention and that she had scheduled me an appointment with a doctor. She wanted me to take anti-depressants. I went to the doctor and was totally pissed off. I was quiet and argumentative with him. My mom told him how I acted. "Fuck these people. They are against me." I thought. He wrote me a prescription for Paxil. I went ahead and took 'em since I had them. Shit, I was feeling a little better, but missed my old self and I resisted feeling overly happy. I began to feel comfortable in my depressed sullen self and thought of myself as a profound heavy thinker. I felt secure walking around in my capsule; my cloud of unhappiness. I quit taking them. There was a new person emerging and I didn't quite know how to handle, the person I remember slightly from middle school.

So, if one tends to be depressed, there are things out there that will make you undepressed and it is like a diabetic who needs insulin. Depression is not physical, it is a psychosis. Though it can be as lethal as a physical situation.

Well this went on for years. On meds, off meds. Up and down. Till I entered university. I finally totally nutted up there. Isolated scribbling in my notepad, broke, struggling with two jobs where I had to be social against my will. I had a manic break. I ended up in a mental hospital for a month. There were five attendants that held me down and injected me with Haldol. Knocked me on my ass for days. This has happened to me four times in my life. They finally diagnosed me with Manic-Depression and finally got me on the right meds—ones I take religiously now.

My prescription to you is: write, read, play with dogs, meds, camp, work, get creative, find a passion, express youself in some form. Smoke pot and listen to Bob Marley on occasion, see the movie *Marley*, go for walks. It is up to you to decide which people are worthy of interacting with you, cause there are interesting people out there who have something to say. As a human with different experiences we actually have something to share. We have to work to have money. We have to deal with many situations. Use you creativity, your knowledge to untangle the situation, to diffuse it. Or carry on a relationship of some kind with the ones you choose, cause you have the power, believe it or not, to choose.

If you work in retail like me, for the past twenty five years, you get to know types of people. Don't judge them because some might surprise you and it will make your day. Hang in there, each day brings something new and different. There are small miracles that happen and savor them. Look for and seek the good in people. Seek the good in yourself because we were chosen, not asked to be on this fucking planet. We might as well take command of our existence and live the way we choose. Things may look grim but this planet keeps on spinning and we are here to create our own purpose. Find it, seek it, keep criticizing, keep feeling blue but find its source—explore your past situations and get them out in some form. Learn from them and don't dwell on them.

Move on and grow from them. Be smarter than your situation. Do something different.

I explored Korea , Yellowstone national park, Thailand, Japan. I didn't have the money to hop in a car or plane, I worked in these places. In Korea for a year teaching the English language, which you can do if you have a college degree in anything. You can go not only to Korea, but anywhere in the world. I was in Yellowstone for the summer, cleaning rooms.

Put yourself in uncomfortable situations and odds are they will turn out better than expected. You meet people along the way experiencing similar situations as you. Learn, grow, reinvent. Everything is temporary. We only consume a small space on the planet—make small steps, then leap. Keep it humble, keep it real. You will emerge a sunflower looming, reaching for the sun and you will create and invent your existence.

BICYCLE COMMUTING

Robert Earl Sutter III

People operating cars behave like they are half human and half machine. With so much attention focused on the operation of this machine, we become a part of it. The act of sitting in that seat and working those controls takes a bit of our humanity away. Sealed in this bubble we cannot hear people on the outside, our visibility is reduced and we cannot see as well, and most important—we can drive a car much faster than our human legs can move. This reduces our reaction time to a dangerous level. We are unable to maintain the vital level of focus all the time while driving. Our interactions with other cyborgs and pedestrians can be reduced to a fight or flight response that is devoid of compassion. It is the technology of the car itself which makes our streets hostile, not necessarily the attitude of the driver. Even a saint driving a car is easily a potential killer.

Recently I was hit by a minivan while it was making an illegal U-turn. I was lucky to see it coming. Other people on the sidewalk saw it coming too. I heard them scream. I braked and turned away from the van, then at the last second I leapt from my bike and hit the ground running, not stopping until I was on the sidewalk. My bike lay under the front end of the van. That could have been it. Right there.

I've been hit by several cars while riding a bicycle. The worst of which involved crashing into a car while riding the wrong way on the sidewalk of a one-way street. I broke my collar bone and it was a lesson learned the hard way. Always have good brakes! Keep your bike in good repair. You only get one body. If you break it, the fun goes away.

Counter-intuitive as it may seem at times, the safest way to ride your bike is to ride in the same direction as the flow of traffic in the same lane with the cars. Ride in a straight line so you are predictible and visible at all times. Keep about three to five feet from the row of parked cars in case someone opens a door suddenly. Other than biking on the sidewalk or against the flow of traffic, intersections and people opening their car doors without looking cause the most bicycle accidents.

I have survived all my bicycling experiences. I have learned to keep my eyes moving, always scanning left to right because every car, every driveway, and every intersection is potential damage and death. At night I use lights with rechargeable batteries in the front and in back. We must stay vigilant on our bikes to give the cyborgs all the help they can get to avoid hitting us. Some of these speeding cyborgs are also intoxicated. Always keep your top eye open. Bicycle riding is an attentive meditation. Stay in the present moment, be mindful of every detail around you: the sounds, movements, lights. The whisper of danger on the wind. Don't test your guardian angels. Be safe, ride free.

PREGNANCY
Kaycee

....

Adelaide would have been born in late August.

A child of New Orleans, she would have braved hot asphalt and mosquitos, cooled herself under warped ceiling fans on splintery paint-peeled porches. She would have found beauty in twinkling tuba brass and flaking sunburns, stubbed her small pink toes on cypress roots and tarmac.

But Adelaide will not join us on ramblings through the swamps of Lafitte Park or for snoballs on the levee. No oyster tongue will be stained a brilliant blue. I decided that Adelaide should be what could have been, and not what will be. Though the decision was the right one, and the healthy choice, I continue to struggle to embrace the decision, and to release the idea of her.

I felt something amiss long before I peed on a little plastic stick. My body felt thick and ponderous, my breasts heavy against my skin, ocean currents moving along my abdomen. After one week, two glasses of wine and my last chewed fingernail, I announced, "I am going to get a pregnancy test." My fiancée, John, looked at me, cautious, unsure of his words. Neither of us knew what to say, so the silence hung delicately between us, a web of uncertainty.

I rented a movie and made dinner. I peed on the stick, I watched it flame up astoundingly within seconds, irrevocably pink slashed—an affront to my status quo. I walked to the kitchen, brought the plates to the table, took a long draught of wine, and announced, "I'm pregnant. I am going to Planned Parenthood tomorrow." John nodded his assent, stunned.

We ate. We watched a movie I can't remember, The ocean in my stomach rumbled until I quelled it with alcohol and eddying tears that would not come. I woke up at 4 am and vomited wine and kale into the toilet bowl, watched it swirl and stared at the gaping space that remained. I was overcome.

The gore-splattered corpse of my parent's marriage left an open wound on my insides—I swore from a young age that childbearing was not for me. Even the word—childbearing—brought unwilling saliva to my mouth. The bloated stomachs of sappy, grinning mothers, needlessly populating an earth overflowing with unwanted, pock-marked babies. The sticky fingers and commercialism. The demands of economy and lifestyle. The impending doom of my parents fondling and cooing, ready to fuck up yet another generation.

When I became a teacher, this feeling intensified, as I watched the children straggling into my room, unloved, uncared for, and so terrifyingly, bitterly angry. I gave them every precious ounce of snuggling ability I had.

John and I bonded immediately over this, along with our shared vegetarianism. We would not be participating in the proverbial circle of life—either with the death of animals for food or the act of procreation.

Planned Parenthood didn't take long to verify what my whole dilated, aching body confirmed—I was pregnant. They made John wait in the waiting room until they confirmed that he would not be coercing me into any decisions—that I wasn't abused. That this is their first step—a private conversation with the woman alone—speaks violent volumes to how women are treated in this country, and I cried for all of these conversations, all of these women, all of these little balls of tissue and cells and blood and pulsing potential.

Normally quick to tears, I kept them in for 24 hours. But here, for the first time, I cried for the simple, fierce need to have it out.

After a brief counseling session, I made an appointment for the only abortion clinic in New Orleans. The few straggling protesters held cardboard signs limply in the winter sunshine— they looked bedraggled and uncared for, stray dog antagonists. Fifteen other women joined me in the waiting room, including another teacher and a former student, who I fortunately spotted before she spotted me and I was quickly smuggled into a backroom to wait until she left—the horrifying dichotomy of wanting to comfort and touch her, the withering fear and shame of being seen in this cement-walled building with its single-minded purpose. The women displayed their various classes— a plastic Wal-mart grocery bag, Gucci high heels tapping, half sewn weave—all sharing tissue and granola bars, sniffling and flipping through tattered magazines.

I signed the paperwork requesting not to hear the heartbeat. I bore the beeping, the Christain disdain and disapproving looks from nurses. I took the sealed envelope containing the only picture that would ever be taken of Adelaide—a little black smudge in a sea of smudges, her existence little more than hope and wasted ink.

Opting for a medical abortion, rather than a surgical one felt more natural and more in line with my mental health. The idea of a vacuum near my uterus made me grey behind the eyes, nauseous. I rented a pile of movies and gathered boxes of tissues. John, attentive and kind, brought me hot toddies and heating pads, and our three pit bulls piled up close on the couch with me, sensing that I needed their warm weight and oven breath.

The first pill is taken at the clinic—the second sets over two days. I bled the existence of Adelaide out, cramps wrenching the occasional whimpers from me, eating cold fruit and pain pills, blood clots and gore dampening the inside of my thighs.

It was a sweaty nightmare, physically draining, I ached from the heart-side out. If I was blessed in one way, it was with a partner who cared for and comforted me, gave me space and listened when I needed it. Most of the women who joined me between those cement walls would brave these days alone. Afterwards, I felt hollow, viscously sad, and free.

Adelaide was not a health issue, in the physical sense. She was not a nuisance. And she was not a liability—John and I could have financially cared for her. We could have raised her on the best books and delicious vegan food, taught her to wrangle pit bulls and gardens and cicadas and syntax and chicks. She could have healed the wounds left upon me by rape and divorce and a life of hard struggle. That she may have leeched these poisons from me made the decision to let her go hardest for both John and I.

But the truth remains that, while I would have demanded that her existence meet these expectations and more, I had little to offer her in return. As much as I wanted to love her, she was not wanted. I cringe to write that, but it's simply true. Making a decision between my mental health, the health of my relationship, and the stability of the life John and I struggled so hard to build—simply was not a choice at all.

I'm forever sorry, Adelaide. And while I will always regret your loss, I will never mourn the choice.

AFTER DRUG ABUSE
Tiffany Roberts

I went through years using hard drugs. The result was a period of panic attacks that left me agoraphobic; afraid to fly, afraid to talk to people, afraid to sleep for fear I would die. It crushed my soul and left me the opposite of myself. I allowed my fear and self-doubt to control my entire existence.

I grew weary of being terrified and sought therapy, both in a clinical setting and on my own with books and cassettes. I needed to be brave or I would lose myself. A few months later I stepped onto an airplane and within a year I was on a stage. From time to time the feelings would still creep out of their caves and tap me on the shoulder, but I refused to turn around. They come less and less each year, the more I ignore them.

You alone hold the power to allow yourself to be dragged into the murky depths of self-doubt, self-loathing, and other thoughts that destroy who you are. Hold your head high. Take control of your life. Be fearless.

Keep a positive attitude despite any challenges tossed your way. Lemons can be turned into lemonade. I find humor in literally every situation in life. Try it; I swear it works.

"Things turn out best for the people who make the best of the way things turn out." —John Wooden

The worst thing you can do for your health is allowing yourself to be treated poorly despite the fact that you are worth everything. This includes how you treat yourself. Surround yourself with positive influences and positive experiences. Cultivate a positive self-image and you will make healthy decisions.

At the same time, it is our right for all people to be safe in the street and to have a family and to be with our loved ones on their deathbed. We should never accept anything less and having the self-confidence makes these struggles for equal rights for all people feel more manageable.

While I was raised in a fairly encouraging environment, support was given more easily for accomplishments that followed a pre-approved path; for those which didn't, proof of success was needed before approval was given. The solidarity and support I receive from GLBTQQA communities, family and friends is perhaps the greatest asset for my health. I have yet to find a community more supportive of my individuality and whole person. We are here for each other. I am cut from a different cloth than my immediate family and thusly needed to look outside it for role models. You are never alone. I guarantee your support, role models, and your muses are out there.

Grasping each opportunity in life as the universe presents it to you, figuratively and sometimes literally, leaping off the pony to grab that brass ring. Never be content to watch when you could be doing. Absorb and appreciate every little thing life has to offer.

BRAIN DAMAGE
Synthia Nicole

At 27 years old I was living in residential rehabilitation for adults with disabilities. I felt fortunate to have shelter, water, and food, and to live in a country that takes care of its disabled with government benefits such as social security disability income (which I'm on). I'm lucky to reside in a country which I have no immediate desire to flee or emigrate from.

My experience of being diagnosed with Arteriovenous Malformations, a kind of brain damage caused by defects of the circulatory system, would likely be different than anyone else's because different parts of the brain would be affected, they would have a different recovery process, they would receive different medication, different chemical balances, or any number of other circumstances.

But still, there is advice that applies to almost anyone. Riding a bicycle and exercising regularly maintain both my physical and mental health. Gardening helps tremendously. Planting and sharing extra for my neighbors and friends is an added bonus.

I do my best not to participate in gossip, even though I do listen to it a bit at work, I mostly don't want to hear it.

I've improved my critical thinking skills because I felt they needed it. I was comparing myself to others, based on their DIY success, friends, social work, scholarly success, or even comparing my physical body. Realizing this has forced me to become more honest and humble. I accepted that my cognitive difficulties limit what and how much I can learn. I'm doing what I enjoy at the moment, even if that's just a nap or removing myself from an environment so I may decompress. I've found that being honest with myself about what I want or need is difficult but the most rewarding.

Being honest with my pain psychologist was much easier. He hadn't witnessed seventeen years of active alcoholism, mood-altering substance disease, and addiction.

By my third time landing in rehab, it was suggested that I should admit to my primary care physician that I am an alcoholic. This was scary, because after my brain injury in 2004, my physician had been there for me when no one else could figure out why I was experiencing pain.

Even after the inflammation had decreased, which was the cause of the constant pain, the process had become an experiment for me. You see, my physician had been hooking me up with narcotics for years. I didn't want them to know I was an alcoholic because, for one reason, he wouldn't continue prescribing narcotics to me so freely, if ever again.

I called the county to ask about substance assistance and was asked who my physician was. I answered and was told that they had recently resigned. What a relief. It was a chance to start over.

When the time came to find new medical support I felt an empowerment in being open and honest about all aspects of my health. I found a new primary physician, a psychologist, and a psychiatrist who all know of my brain injury, disability, alcoholism, and recovery. Surprisingly, four months after I quit using mood-altering substances, my chronic pain became more manageable.

Prior to my brain injury I was vegan. I was employed by a naturopath in a vegan, organic, raw food restaurant. I ate fruits, vegetables, legumes, and grains. I also ingested lots of Old Style beer and whatever other alcohol was on hand.

Nine years later, I now eat what feels good, which currently includes a good amount of dark chocolate.

I mull over my choices carefully now. I'm aware that I don't always make the best decisions, sometimes due to my brain injury, but now I consult with others and take some time to make my choices.

I don't regret my past; it's gotten me where I am. But I don't look into the future that much either. I plan ahead, like planning to stay in Nashville with a friend and their child this summer. I want to make a trip to Dollyworld, so I'm saving money and physical energy for this. But I rarely pass a chance to make a zine with the six year old I live with whenever she wanders into my room. While you can't plan everything to a tee, I plan some days with a rough draft, and the rest with an empty slate.

Synthia Nicole writes and publishes Damaged Mentality *zine and can be reached at: sydny77@gmail.com or www.wemakezines.ning/profile/chinagirl*

LYME DISEASE

Tasha Van Zandt

I grew up with cabinets stocked full of Little Debbie Snacks and Spaghettio's. But I was also raised with a family that has an outlook on love and happiness as life's greatest teachers.

Four years ago I developed an illness that left me temporally unable to walk or stand. After hospitalization and extensive physical therapy I was able to regain my strength. Although I had enough strength to walk again, a multitude of new and excruciating symptoms had arisen. My case baffled teams of top specialists and the next four years were riddled with visits to top doctors and hospitals where countless numbers of tests and procedures were performed. But not one specialist could find a clear answer and in the summer of 2011 I was hospitalized again. This time I was placed on a strict starvation diet of no water or food due to my system shutting down. I suffered major complications with my heart, lungs, pancreas, liver, gall bladder, and kidneys. The doctors were baffled by my case and after weeks of hospitalization I was sent to the Mayo Clinic to complete months of intensive tests and procedures. The root of my rapidly deteriorating health remained uncertain and I was passed from specialist to specialist.

By some great miracle, my partner referred me to see his Naturopathic Lyme Literate Doctor. I was diagnosed with Lyme Disease and several co-infections. I began intensive injection treatment and natural treatment as well. Within months I was riding my bike and feeling alive again. I began realizing the miracle of treating food as medicine and I learned ways that I can control my health through intention and diet. As cheesy as it is, we really are what we eat. When we are eating natural, organic, sustainable, plant based diets we can be at our healthiest. Being mindful from the ground up allows us to develop a greater awareness of the impact of our choices in all things.

The U.S. food system is causing so many terrible illnesses for the people of our country and yet refuses to change. One in three children born after the year 2000 will suffer from an obesity related illness. The way that our country views food is very compartmentalized and detrimental to our health and our environment.

My health remains a struggle every day. There are days when my legs won't work or my arms are too weak to move. There are days when it feels like I'm trapped in this body. I still have not fully recovered and recently had to go through surgery and several procedures. But the change is that there are more days when I feel acceptance, peace, and hope.

Life is impermanent. Therefore, everything else is too. By being mindful of the impermanence we can let go of the past and the future and be mindful of the moment. Even though it may be a difficult moment, it is simply a moment. I wouldn't be where I am today if it weren't for the struggles I've been through. When we get carved away by our struggles, the strongest parts remain and shine through at their brightest.

Spending time with my best friend and partner, Sebastian, makes me feel my absolute happiest. Learning from people makes my heart full. I feel lucky to have so many people that make me feel this way. Creating things makes me feel full as well, like creating art, singing songs, playing in the sunshine, and cooking good food with good people.

Mindfulness of my loved ones, my surroundings, and myself has been one of the most powerful things in my life. When we think in mindful and holistic ways about ourselves and our environments we naturally make healthy and compassionate choices.

It's really difficult not to worry in life. Except worry won't do anything for the future while it ruins your present. One of my favorite quotes is:

"I am an old man and have known a great many troubles, but most of them have never happened." —Mark Twain

Tasha Van Zandt founded a Photovoice project called LymeVoice to promote awareness of Lyme Disease. www.lymevoice.weebly.com You can view Tasha's artwork at www.natatashavanzandt.com

NERVOUS BREAKDOWN

Sandra Fragola

Last year, I suffered a nervous/mental breakdown while dealing with multiple crises. The loss of two important relationships (one with a bisexual man and one with a dyke) was one crisis of many. Together it created a snowball effect.

Sanity slipped through my fingers. My doctor prescribed anti-psychotic medication for stress and anxiety but I didn't disclose my breakdown out of fear. The thought of seeing a psychiatrist sickened me and I was worried about being locked up. Instead, I placed myself in the hands of supportive, non-judgemental atmosphere with a psychotherapist, which put my life into perspective.

Taking care of my mental health became a priority and I had to think of ways to eliminate destructive thought patterns from my life, which is still ongoing. If I thought something "bad" would happen if I cut my hair, I fought those thoughts and shaved my head. With a razor.

Meeting people and socializing was one of many big obstacles to overcome. It was terrifying and at the same time, depressing. I'm still trying to find ways to break the ice. I am still learning to take care of myself and be nurturing. I didn't think I'd get through what happened but I've come a long way since my breakdown. I'm still in therapy, thinking about weaning off my meds.

I'm becoming more artistic, creative, and productive. There are still areas of my life I need to work through. But life is a process and I'm still getting to know myself. Learning not to be self-destructive and being aware that if I am self-destructive remains a big challenge in my life. Fortunately, I love a challenge and refuse to allow a major mental health issue to hold me down. My life has been steered in the right direction. And I'm looking forward to achieving my goals and not settling for less than what I deserve.

A DAY IN MY WHEELS
BY JANIS DIAZ

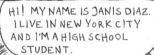

HI! MY NAME IS JANIS DIAZ. I LIVE IN NEW YORK CITY AND I'M A HIGH SCHOOL STUDENT.

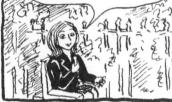

I HAVE OSTEOGENISIS IMPERFECTA, SOMETIMES CALLED "BRITTLE BONE DISEASE." THAT MEANS MY BONES ARE VERY FRAGILE, AND IT'S WHY I'M IN A WHEEL CHAIR.

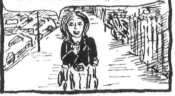

A LOT OF PEOPLE HAVE NO IDEA OF WHAT IT IS LIKE TO LIVE WITH A DISABILITY, SO THAT'S WHAT I WANT TO GET AT — A DAY IN MY WHEELS.

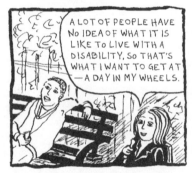

RIGHT NOW I'M IN A PARK AND THERE'S A CUTE GUY ON A BENCH ACROSS FROM ME. EXCUSE ME, WOULD YOU EVER DATE A DISABLED GIRL?

HUH?

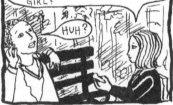

I KNOW IT SOUNDS LIKE I'M COMING ON TO YOU, BUT I'M MAKING A RADIO DOCUMENTARY. WOULD YOU EVER DATE A DISABLED GIRL?

IF SHE'S LIKE YOU...

I'LL GET YOUR NUMBER LATER.

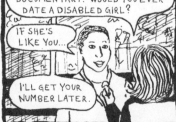

SOME PEOPLE THINK IF YOU'RE DISABLED, YOU'RE NOT INTERESTED IN CERTAIN TYPES OF RELATIONSHIPS. BUT HEY, I'M DISABLED — I'M NOT A NUN.

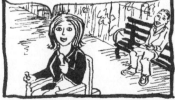

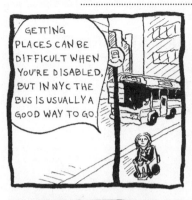

GETTING PLACES CAN BE DIFFICULT WHEN YOU'RE DISABLED, BUT IN NYC THE BUS IS USUALLY A GOOD WAY TO GO.

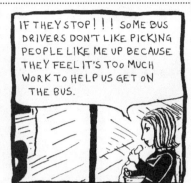

IF THEY STOP!!! SOME BUS DRIVERS DON'T LIKE PICKING PEOPLE LIKE ME UP BECAUSE THEY FEEL IT'S TOO MUCH WORK TO HELP US GET ON THE BUS.

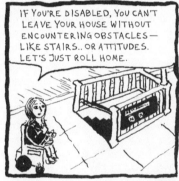

IF YOU'RE DISABLED, YOU CAN'T LEAVE YOUR HOUSE WITHOUT ENCOUNTERING OBSTACLES — LIKE STAIRS.. OR ATTITUDES. LET'S JUST ROLL HOME.

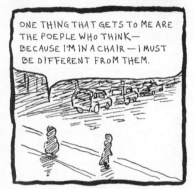

ONE THING THAT GETS TO ME ARE THE POEPLE WHO THINK — BECAUSE I'M IN A CHAIR — I MUST BE DIFFERENT FROM THEM.

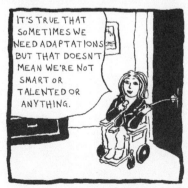

IT'S TRUE THAT SOMETIMES WE NEED ADAPTATIONS BUT THAT DOESN'T MEAN WE'RE NOT SMART OR TALENTED OR ANYTHING.

THERE'S A BOY I KNOW WHO HAS SCARS FROM HIS SURGERIES. I TOLD HIM HIS SCARS SHOW HE'S BEEN THROUGH WAR, AND THAT HE'S BRAVE AND STRONG. THESE SCARS ARE PART OF WHO WE ARE. I WOULDN'T TRADE MY DISABILITY TO BE LIKE OTHER PEOPLE. THIS IS JANIS DIAZ.

THIS IS AN EXCERPT FROM <u>YO, MISS — A GRAPHIC LOOK AT HIGH SCHOOL</u> BY LISA WILDE. IT IS BASED ON INTERVIEWS WITH JESSICA DE LA ROSA.

BREAST CANCER
Rachel Morgan

Dear World,
I send news that the cancer did not metastasize and the drudgery is mostly over. It's been an enlightening battle over the last 6 ½ weeks to naturally draw out the tumor from my breast. While it's been the longest, most painful six weeks of my life, I'm feeling better. I've been humbled by the process, waking up every two hours from pain, not eating, rotating the same couple pairs of pajama's for 45 days, not being able to shower, and having my mother scrub the hard to reach places of my back during sponge bath time only gives me a hope of a bright future. And I discovered it is possible to fall asleep on my hands and knees while making jewelry or surfing the internet on the floor.

I had this breast tumor with me for 6 years in this life. So I chose a non-invasive procedure that my natural practitioner suggested a few years back. It is a way to have the body eliminate the tumor without a lumpectomy or mastectomy. I used this product called Amazon Black Salve made of bloodroot, chaparral, and zinc chloride in which I apply topically to the breast skin area of the tumor and take small amounts internally. The Black Salve goes after neoplastic (cancerous) tissue, breaking down the tumor membrane. Then the immune system pushes the neoplasm through the breast tissue to the surface of the skin, forms an eschar and detaches through the skin. Wow, I feel like I should be on a Science TV Show for kids!

I kept my pH balance in the high alkaline range. Tumors cannot grow in an alkaline environment, only in an acidic one, so changing to and maintaining a high pH is crucial to stop the radical cell growth. I did reflexology treatments every four days with my natural practitioner keeping my immune system in tip-top shape. We also did emotional release therapy to liberate and heal the anger and fear that caused the tumor to form in the first place. And I've learned that in order to heal the body, I had to release the pain and memories that I was holding onto in my heart to rid the cause of the ailment. You've got to let go, forgive yourself and others. Basically, I can walk on water now.

After 45 days, the tumor, now named Toomz, has eliminated through the surface of my skin. The last two weeks were the worst. I couldn't remember what life was like before I started the elimination process. Trying to be funny and helpful, my father suggested we put maggots on the fleshy wound to eat the dead tissue as they did before modern medicine. He was 50% serious. Once you are on the ferris wheel you must stay on the ferris wheel until the ride is over, even if you are screaming, crying, and vomiting while Randy the Carny leaves the ride with three underage girls to smoke a big joint in his trailer.

There were times I wished I had gotten conventional surgery. But *everyone* does that. Sometimes they come out unscathed, but usually minus a breast and with all the cells in their body irradiated. I like the Hocus Pocus Voodoo Warrior way. Or I thought I would try it. Now my breast should heal up with minor scarring and I eliminated the cancer in a short time compared to modern medicine. But I can't take all the credit: I could not have done it without the help of prescription pain medication. I had Vicodin, Codeine, and Morphine at my bedside in case the waves of pain reached the unbearable level, which they often did.

I consider myself a person who can endure hardship but this pain was out of control. I never slept and toward the end, the pill bottles were getting empty, so I had to start rationing pain meds. I would wait out the pain all day until it was time to clean the wound in the evening. I never want to ration again.

But what am I going to do now? Run for the next Presidential election? Create new flavors of Ben and Jerry's ice cream? Be on a Girls Gone Wild segment to flash my clean bill of health breast for the world to see? As attractive as all those ideas sound, I can't wait to get back to dancing, drinking wine, and eating exotic meals. For now, I am going to take a 47-minute shower then sleep in a wide array of positions other than on my back.

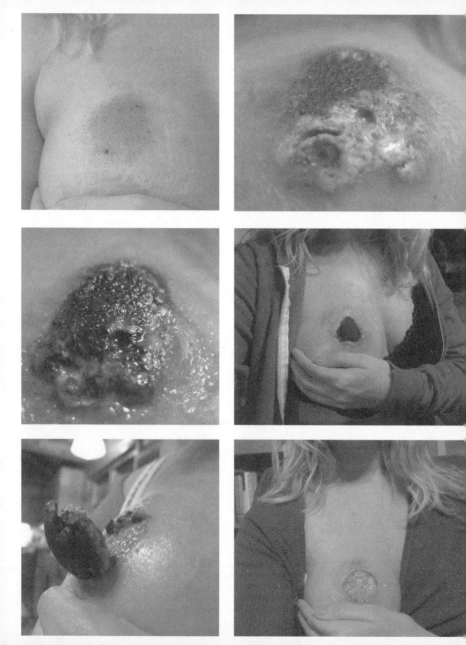

DOCTOR INTERNET AND THE COLLECTIVE CONSCIOUSNESS

Robert Earl Sutter III

I have been consulting the collective consciousness, accessed through the internet, for my health needs for years. Studying a diverse selection of postings and comments about a particular subject can bring you to a mean average of understanding—superior sometimes to even an expert's knowledge. The collective is wiser than the individual, after you average out the extreme points of view. This phenomenon can be explained in a real story about a street fair where random folks were asked to judge the weight of a cow. They each wrote down their answers. A scientist collected the pieces of paper and discovered that the average of all the guesses was almost the perfect weight of the cow, coming even closer to the exact weight than the individual experts on cows who were present.

This information is exciting. We have evolved to be this way: a group of altruistic people, not a group of selfish individuals. The group that cares about the individuals triumphs over a group who focus on their individual wants and needs. We love heroes, people who sacrifice themselves for the greater good. We like these people, they guarantee that our groups survive evolution.

Western medicine does not share knowledge or power in the same way. U.S. drug companies do most of the research and development for new drugs that are used across the globe and are paid for through inflated prices in the U.S. Because the lifetime and profitability of a drug is often unknown and prices will need to be lower in much of the world, the cost in the U.S. is maximized, especially for people who have insurance that will pay the inflated price. The medical establishment can hold the power of life and death over us in a hierarchic system, but the decisions about our life should be our own.

Recently, I found a lump on my knee and was experiencing increasing pain in the joint, so I went to a doctor, got an MRI scan, and the doctor diagnosed it as a Meniscus Tear with the lump being a result, a Meniscus Cyst. "We will schedule you for an arthroscopy," the doctor said before ending the visit.

The doctor hadn't even described what an arthroscopy was. I consulted the internet and learned what the surgery entailed. My partner found an article about Meniscus Tears and I found out that 70% of people with a torn meniscus respond to physical therapy as a remedy with the same results as an arthroscopy, but without the unnecessary surgery and possible risks. I was pissed!

An arthroscopy costs more than twice as much as physical therapy does. I canceled the surgery and I won't be going back to that doctor. Now every day I do Hamstring Curls, Heel Dig Bridging, Toe Raises, Quad Stretches, Straight Leg Raise To The Back, Straight Leg Raise To The Front. After only a few days I noticed a change, the pain was going away. Wow.

The power to heal myself was there all along. Always trust yourself and get a second opinion from your friend.

Paralysis of Fear

Nathan Lee Thomas

I exited the streetcar, running late for work, and attempted to make it to a connecting bus at a dead sprint and pulled a muscle or tore a tendon so badly it had me inching my way up the sidewalk, leaning on the sides of buildings in a slow crawl to fight back the pain. I sometimes sit with only one cheek on my office chair and the other extended straight out or standing up at my desk and leaning over in order to find some relief from the multilayered pain which travels all the way from the heel of my right foot to my knee, hip, lower back, neck, and temple.

Over the years I've been forced to visit several specialists about this at the urgings and insistence of others who had my best interests in mind, I'm sure, but none of the doctors or other medical professionals I met with could nail down with any certainty the cause or source of my pain and I was met with every imaginable response from being told I was wasting their time and how they only treated people with real emergencies to the time the doctor insinuated I was only interested in the pain pills and refused treatment, assuming I was a drug addict. Others prescribed medical shoe insoles or a bulky nighttime brace, which would keep my foot bent to prevent my tendon from shortening.

A wonderful massage therapist would tug and pull, hook me up to an electric shock muscle relaxer, leave the room for ten minutes, then go to work on smoothing out the bumps. But it would just provide some temporary relief and as soon as I left the office, the pain returned. I thought that perhaps my right leg was shorter than the other and maybe I should invest in something to even them out. But the massage therapist said it was too dramatic and my body wouldn't be able to handle it after all these years.

It seemed as though everything I believed to be a perfectly logical and rational question or observation was met with the same kind of dismissal. It was as if I was telling them how to do their job. They were the experts and I was the uneducated, inexperienced one who should keep quiet while they worked their magic. When I told the foot doctor, who prescribed four-hundred-dollar insoles, about how much bigger the largest toe on my right foot was than the left, he dismissed it with a carefully-prepared statement about how this was common in most people and not to worry about it.

I wasn't just worried about the length of my right leg or the size of my big toe. It worried me that whenever I attempted to offer suggestions or lead any of them in another direction they moved in the opposite direction. Was it simply out of some deep-seated sense of entitlement which came with their stature in society? Why couldn't I just follow their directions and keep my mouth shut? It was as if they were taking my questions and comments personally, felt threatened or challenged by them, and needed to go in another direction just to show who was in charge. It caused me to become even more suspicious of them and their "good" intentions.

Every conversation and dismissal reminded me of something my mother had told me years earlier, without a medical degree. Preceded by me running up to her, explaining how contorting some part of my body into an unnatural configuration hurt, she would explain, in the simplest motherly medical advice, "Well, if it hurts when you do that, then stop doing it, silly."

And like magic, she was right. It would immediately stop hurting every time.

So, I began to wonder: What did all these pains have in common? What did all of these individual remedies from several different medical professionals and their expert advice have in common? I began a personal quest to discover the solution on my own using the missing ingredient my mother had provided so many years before.

Since then I've managed to live a relatively pain free life for years without another single visit to any more of these high-priced experts.

The first thing I did was put out my feelers. I became acutely aware of every single twinge or ache in my entire body and what immediately preceded it and what, if anything, I was able to do to prevent this activity in the future. I used medical practices I observed during my doctor visits, like the way they would look for differences between the right side of my body and the the left. I noticed something remarkable about two things which stood out significantly to me and attempted to revisit two things which had always bothered me from when I first began to experience all of this pain.

Why not see if I can address these issues with the right side of my body, since this was the side experiencing all the pain and my left was not. What was different? How was I going to try and make them the same?

So I began experimenting with one extra insole in my right shoe, then two, and three, and back down, until I found a reduced level of pain. To my surprise it worked!

Then I moved to this annoying big toe of mine and something else became abundantly clear. When I would look down at my bare feet and bend my toes, I noticed my left foot would create a perfectly perpendicular line with the rest of my foot without pain. However, when I bent my right foot in the same manner, my unnaturally large toe would force my foot to bend at a forty-five degree angle. This had a ripple effect on the rest of my body to the point that my entire right leg was forced to bow outward in such a manner that it was shortening my leg.

I was astonished! I was on to something here!

Then I remembered the overnight foot brace they gave me to keep my ankle from straightening out. Could my toe's inability to bend be causing similar effects? Perhaps the same principle applied and it was not only my ankle straightening overnight, but my right toe's refusal to bend all day long which was contributing to this shortening effect!

Then I remembered the doctor who had refused to treat me because he only treated people with real foot problems and how I was wasting his time. Something I explained to him before he blew me off was that the boots I was wearing completely eliminated my pain for the first few months I wore them. My pain only returned after the heels of the shoes had began to wear more on the outside than the inside, creating an unnatural rocking motion with an outward lean or bowed walk.

Were the new boots, with their over-sized soles that went beyond the width of my heel, preventing my right toe from pushing my leg into an outward bow and correcting my walk?

Then I had my epiphany. This stupid toe of mine was creating a chain reaction, which extended all the way from my heel to my neck. It was preventing my foot from bending at that crucial point. It was shortening my tendons and muscles, causing pain in my heel. It was shortening my leg by bowing it outward, causing unnatural force against my knee and hip. It was throwing my back out as well, by causing me to change my walk. I would prevent my right heel from landing flat on the ground, and overuse the muscles on the right side of my body to compensate.

Something had to be done.

So, after much deliberation and even more attempts to find the perfect solution through a thoughtful process of elimination and lots of trial and error, I was able to come up with the following solution I still use to this day.

I stretch my legs every night before I go to sleep and throughout the day, concentrating on the big toe by bending it back as much and as often as possible. I place an extra thin insole inside my right shoe to compensate for my right leg's insistence on shortening, but mostly I do everything in my power to prevent this shortening in the first place by forcing my big toe to bend and keep it from bowing my leg out. I create a more natural gait through brute force.

Having multiple doctors offer insufficient solutions and refuse to treat my pain tested my determination, but my frustrations gave me the courage to seek my own solution. It takes most of my concentration and makes it difficult to walk and chew gum at the same time, but it is a step towards achieving a permanent and lasting cure. ...or something like that.

The only thing it couldn't remedy was my insistence on waiting until the last possible minute to head out the door on my way somewhere. I'm still running at a dead sprint after connecting buses. The important difference now is I can do it with confidence and, dare I say it again? Vigor!

HEADGEAR
Anna Ricklin

On the advice of our family dentist, my parents took me to an orthodontist when I was six years old. He told them my mouth was too small for all of my teeth. He said I needed to have some teeth extracted to make room for others. So began ten years of oral torture.

So, at the age of six, just after my two front teeth had grown in, I had eight baby teeth pulled out. When I was eight, I had four more; and when I was ten, he took four permanent adult teeth—pre-molars—all in the name of making space in my mouth to create the perfect smile. What this doctor did, of course, was to violently interrupt my growth and intervene in one of the most intimate parts of the human body, creating an imbalance that hurt. At the age of six, I was initiated into a world of chronic pain originating in my head, and for which I can only treat the symptoms.

I remember sitting down in the surgeon's chair the first time, a little girl with two long braids, wanting to please her parents and not really understanding what was about to happen. The gas mask over my face, the terrible sticky smell, and a vision of an elastic band spinning faster and slower against a blood red background. It is one of the most startling and unpleasant things to awaken groggy, unable to move properly, and bleeding from the mouth. Rather than waiting for my teeth naturally to fall from my mouth, they were taken. And then it happened twice more. I do not understand why my parents allowed it to happen again, let alone twice, but they thought they were doing the best for me. I followed, because it never occurred to me that there was another option. I never said no.

In between the tooth extractions I had braces, a palette expander, and headgear. Even though this was the 1980s, the devices of modern orthodonture at that time were barbaric. Whatever balance that could have been found despite the violent taking of teeth was then made impossible by literally changing the shape of my mouth by force. The pallet expander fit into the roof of my mouth. Every two days someone—usually one of my parents but sometimes the nurse at school—inserted a little "key" into a screw in the apparatus and turn it, pushing outwards on the bone and thus widening my hard pallet. The headgear, by contrast, was an external device, an arc of stainless steel that fit into two metal bands on my back molars, protruding from my face and making it difficult to sleep on my side. I'm still not sure of its exact purpose, but the discomfort caused by both of these contraptions—not to mention the tearing of my lips and gums by braces and the pulling of miniature rubber bands—called upon all of the New England stoicism instilled in me from a young age. I said nothing, but once I did bite the doctor pretty hard.

I had braces twice. The first time, from age 8-10. At the age of 12 they came back for four more years. My existence included regular visits to the orthodontist to get my braces tightened, a band replaced, to lie in the chair with my mouth open and hands reaching in. I steeled myself. Mostly it was just part of life, but like most children, I didn't know that it could be changed or stopped.

Around the time I turned 16—just before my junior year of high school, and before my braces came off—I started to notice that my jaw felt out of place. It didn't open or close smoothly and it started to hurt. I noticed that when I closed my mouth it wasn't comfortable to rest my top and bottom teeth together, like they didn't fit right. We went to the doctor, who of course proposed a whole new set of procedures to "treat" this new problem, called TMJ (the letters simply stand for the name of the joint: tempor-mandibular joint, the place where the mandible articulates with the temporal bones of the skull). This time, I pulled back. I didn't want this person in my mouth any more. When my braces were finally removed in the spring of my junior year, I got my retainers and didn't go back. But the damage was done. I have suffered from TMJ for 18 years, and there is no way to truly fix the disorder. As with so many things joint-related, the injury leaves a permanent impression.

By the time I ended college and entered my early 20s, my TMJ was so painful that it was a distraction. I feared the pain and its overwhelming presence in my head. I couldn't eat fun foods like apples or corn on the cob, and it brought headaches too. I couldn't differentiate between my jaw and the rest of my head—the deep aching all blended together. Still, my New England stoicism prevailed most of the time, and I didn't complain or seek help as I should have—I didn't know how. The problem only came to the surface on occasions when the pain had been so overwhelming for so many days that I couldn't hold it in anymore and released the hurt with sobs.

This pain contributed to a slow wearing away at my self-confidence, at my sense of place and direction. I thought to myself: "I can't do a full time job with this pain. I couldn't endure graduate school in such agony, I would be too exhausted, too stressed, too worn to succeed." And deep inside I had another fear: "What partner could I find who would want to be with someone like me?"

At some point, though, amidst a crisis of pain, I started to think about how I could overcome the disorder rather than be overwhelmed—and controlled—by it. Now independent from my parents, who had not known how to help me, I started a search to direct my own healing. I discovered yoga in my last year of college and began a regular practice. Yoga helped pull my energy and attention away from my head and connected to the rest of my body. A couple of years later I tried acupuncture to treat the pain, which helped enormously, and then my acupuncturist recommended a chiropractor who worked in a precise and non-invasive approach. The two modalities, together with my yoga practice, helped set my body on a course of self-healing and I started to have days without headaches, without as much jaw pain. I learned how to exercise, which I hadn't done growing up, and focused more and more on what kinds of foods I ate to help reduce inflammation. Later I found an amazing dentist who finally gave me the right kind of mouth guard to wear at night and allow my jaw a rest. As progress happened, I became more motivated to continue.

In the process of seeking care, I learned how to stand up for myself. In fact, I see the whole process of seeking care as an act of standing up for myself. I don't tell my story lying down—I insist on sitting up and looking doctors in the eye. I have invited friends to come with me to new doctors so I have an ally, someone on my side who believes me as I lay out my complaints. While my experience with bad healthcare early in life has made me cynical about the intentions of doctors, I have found caring people to help me take care of myself, mostly outside the dominant medical system. I don't go back to people who do not validate my position and support not only the physical but emotional trauma I have experienced.

As I look back, I would describe the majority of my 20s as a period of searching for healing, for the magic bullet of relief. I know now that no one thing will make me better, or make pain go away, or make me forever balanced in mind and body. For me, it requires a mix of things: exercise, healthy eating, and the support of a handful of good health providers. I have adjusted my budget to allow for healthcare expenses not covered by insurance, which is most of them, and live minimally in other parts of my life. Change has been slow, but I am happy to say that I am more pain free and feel better now, at 34, than I was ten years ago.

Another great thing has come from my experience of chronic pain: I used it to motivate my career. I realized one day that I wanted to help prevent this from happening to other people, to avoid more suffering. When I finally decided to return to school, I studied public health, a field closely related to medicine but aims to stop injury and disease before they occur, rather than treating the effects of illness after they have set in. As a high school or college student, I never would have thought I would be doing something in the field of health, but my passion for my own health helped direct me to turn my pain into my focus—for my benefit.

Living with chronic pain is an ongoing challenge requiring nearly full-time attention, but I have found, carved, and demanded the tools necessary to survive, and I am winning.

DIVORCE

Kirsten Rudberg

I've never felt safe. I've always had one foot out the door, one eye looking behind me, sure that the ground was crumbling behind me, underneath my feet.

By "feeling safe," I mean that feeling where you can let go, breathe deeply and relax, feel good and happy, with no cares in the world. I like to think that I was born feeling this way, feeling safe, that I enjoyed a few years of this bliss, but my parents divorce ended that.

The reason for their divorce wasn't any one thing. I think their unhappiness, and thus mine, began before I can remember. It's always been a family joke that I never smiled in childhood photos. I look at those pictures and wonder why no one noticed. That it became normal for a kid to never smile, never be happy, never feel safe.

I can't entirely blame my parents. As I look at it, they were just two grown-up kids. My Dad was a workaholic and not home a lot, and my Mom felt lonely and overwhelmed by three children. Thus, when my mother had her breakdown and had to go into the mental hospital, my Dad's reaction was that it was "no big deal." And when the judge evicted my Dad from the house and he still came in the back door at his usual time, sat at the table, and ate dinner like nothing was wrong while my Mother raged at the other end, I tried to think the same, "no big deal." Being unbalanced and crazy was the normal for my house. But underneath it all I was forgetting to breathe.

I was the oldest, and my brother and sister were little, too young to understand the hate and anger that happened every day. How is a little girl supposed to understand when her Mom lunges at her Dad with a knife? How is a kindergartner like my brother supposed to deal with the screaming, the fighting, the sobbing? How was I supposed to deal with my Mom, who became depressed and angry, struggling with feeding three kids, working bad jobs to pay the mortgage, while trying to give us lives? How was I supposed to deal with a little brother who started sleep walking every night, and a little sister who stood at the back door crying, begging my father to come back? How was I supposed to deal with the fact there was no solid ground under my feet, that many times I was the adult in the house and that my Mom had decided to "go on strike." I remember the first time she locked her bedroom door. I knew it would be a few days or a week, but either way someone had to keep things going. So I made the dinners, did the laundry, got us to school, and always was holding my breath, waiting, watching, one eye watching the ground crumble apart.

I wanted to leave and escape; to scream at my parents "Stop acting like children!" I wanted my Mom to stop taking it out on me. After my Dad moved out she had no one else to take her anger out on. I was the oldest, and assumed the role of sitting and letting her do her worst. The screaming and the anger didn't happen every day. But I could feel it building. I knew it was a matter of time and I had nowhere to go, so I watched and waited and held my breath. I wanted to feel safe, just once, to relax and be "normal" and still. But it never came. So I held my breath and my words. I kept every little moment of stress, anger, and sadness tightening up inside.

I carry this with me. I carry my sister and brother's pain. I carry my Mother's anger, my Father's disappointment. Because of this I keep one foot out the door, always.

It has not helped me in my life. The stress of both feeling like I'm going forward, but holding back is terrible. I'm scared to date anyone, and if I do, I've got one foot out the door. I'm scared to let people know me because if people get close, they hurt you. They do and say things to wound you, to tear you apart. I'm scared to be vulnerable, because I've only ever had to be strong.

But then I heard a talk by Brene Brown. She said that opening up and being vulnerable is actually being strong, being brave. I thought about my friends and their secrets and how they trusted me with them. I thought about being open, being known better, about breaking open my shell. I thought about how free I would feel if there were some people I could be around and relax, and feel safe. I thought about how free I would feel, and just having that thought made me breathe a little easier.

So I tried it. Baby steps terrified me. Little bits of information helped people know me better. I found that the more I opened up, the greater my friendships, the deeper the connection. I have to consciously swallow and take deep breaths and step forward each day, bring both feet with me, refuse to look behind me, because that is the past. And each day

I leave that past behind, a little more of it falls away. I don't want to be defined by my Mother's anger and depression, I don't want to carry my Father's disappointment and feeling of helplessness. It is day by day. I look forward, to being both strong and vulnerable.

Over time I've realized my parents were just "big kids," with no idea of how to be grown up, how to talk about their fear and sadness. They only knew how to wound and hurt each other—one giant back and forth with no end. Seeing them as people who didn't mean to hurt me, who didn't mean to give me this legacy of sadness and fear, has helped me to forgive them. I'd like to think they've taught me how to be generous and kind, and forgiving, most of all. The other option, to behave like they did, is just not a choice for me.

Its taken years. I tell people that I am a work in progress. It does get better. It just takes time, a whole lot of courage, and remembering to breathe.

ABLATION SALVATION

Lauren Hage

Imagine sitting on the toilet, for hours at a time, waiting and watching as golf ball-sized blood clots fall from between your legs—massaging your lower abdominal to help push out the bigger ones. While having the most painful cramps (not even prescription painkillers or birth control pills helped the level of pain, which I was told by multiple practitioners was comparable to childbirth), cold sweat shakes, and nausea, all at the same time.

I tried using the largest tampons, the thickest pads, and menstrual cups: I would bleed through all of them within an hour or less. Hormonal birth control pills and patches and herbal remedies, all promising to lighten my flow and ease the pain, but nothing worked. They only made my hair fall out, caused rashes and hives, and gave me horrible mood swings. Painkillers that were strong enough to dull the pain slightly made me feel even worse: tight throat, medicine head, and rapid heartbeat scared the shit out of me.

The best I could do was sit on the toilet, push out as much blood as possible, plug up with a super-sized tampon or menstrual cup, place a diaper-sized night pad on my underwear, swallow some aspirin, lay a thick towel on my bed, and pass out from all the pain. I would wake at every hour, lying in a pool of my own blood, get up, and do it all over again.

Dysmenorrhea and Menorrhagia was my life every 28 days, for 6-8 days at a time, for 10 years. There had to be a better way to live. My condition was causing Anemia from all the blood I lost. So I did some research and found out about a non-hormonal, permanent solution, with minimal to no side effects. Endometrial ablation is what I found to best fit my problems,—a procedure that, by means of permanently burning off the lining of my uterus, would stop my periods and fertilized eggs would not have anything to implant into. The trick was to find a doctor that was willing to preform the operation for me. It is normally used for women near menopause and who are finished having children.

I was 25 at the time, living in the Midwest, and did not have or plan to ever have children. This was going to be tricky. Luckily, I stumbled across this wonderful woman doctor eight hours away, who had the record of doing the most ablations in America and was accredited for being the best. I set up the appointment, saved up the thousands of dollars, and I opted for Essure—small metal coils are slipped into the fallopian tubes that cause the body to create a natural barrier with scar tissue, preventing pregnancy. Since I was allergic to condoms (the latex and lube), I needed something so I wouldn't get an ectopic pregnancy.

I was nervous in the waiting room, full of older ladies (including the receptionists) giving me a look of "why is she here?" I was sent back to a set of chairs at the end of a long hallway. A lady with a clipboard asked if I was done having children, I replied, "Yes."

She smiled and said, "Awwww. How many?"

"Zero."

Her immediate reaction was shock, then a fast fade to anger, "What!? Don't you want to have kids?"

"No."

She mumbled something and wrote on my chart. Then she led me to an exam room where I waited for the doctor. The only magazines in the room were about parenting or exercise—which if you think of it, is strange since the only reason women would come here is because they are done with kids, and don't have the energy to workout.

After the usual half-hour wait, the doctor came in. Her winning looks made her seem like she was a model for a doctor on a TV commercial, rather than the actual award-winning intellectual that she was.

I had lots of questions for her; I wanted to know exactly what she would be doing, the side effects, etc. But as I feared, the conversation that took place was me trying to prove that I never wanted to have kids. I got frustrated, but didn't want to loose my chance of getting it done, I had driven all this way, saved up so much money, this *had* to happen. I butted in and told her that if it would make her feel better, I would sign some kind of an agreement that I wouldn't sue her for making me not be able to have kids.

Her reply was, "I'm just concerned about if you find a man and you want to have his kids in the future."

What? On my chart I had put that I *was* with a man, under the question, "What kind of sex partners do you and have you had?" And that we were in a long-term relationship (six years then and still together).

She was embarrassed, "Aren't you a Lesbian? Your chart says "partner'?"

"Yes, my partner is Jeff, he is a man, he is in the waiting room, if you want, you can speak with him."

Her nerve to assume that a *man* would change my mind, now or in the future, was insulting, like my suffering meant nothing—she was so amazed that I was "straight" that she quickly changed the subject of kids, and started to actually talk to me about what it was exactly she would be doing the next day; I passed the consultation. Finally.

I went home with a pill to take that night; it was to dilate my cervix so the instruments could easily fit through, the side effect would be cramps—one last time. The next day I went in and had the preliminary ultrasound, which found cysts on my ovaries, common, but of course painful. The procedure that I was having done wouldn't change that, but I *could* live with that inconvenience.

The nurse gave me a Valium and I went into the room to have the in-clinic operation done. I laid down on a bendable plastic bed with soft pillows and sheets, then the nurse gave me a pair of new fluffy socks to wear to keep my feet warm. It was a souvenir, I suppose, with the clinic's logo on the ankles. Then she hooked up the IV in my arm and turned the lights down low for the medicine to take hold. The IV fluid was of some medicine that had amnesic side effects. That scared me a little, but I figured it was for the best.

Then the doctor came in with 5 nurses to tend to different machines. There was a TV in the corner of the room where I could watch the insides of me through the tiny thin camera that the doctor slid inside me. She first tried inserting the Essure stents. The first one on my right side went in just fine; no pain, no hassle. But the left side didn't want to go in right. I could feel the pricking sensation and see her tweezers trying to place the stubborn last one. She told me that she'd try again after the ablation. She chose the Novasure method. Other methods included a balloon filled with hot water to burn the lining. This new method involved a gold net that expanded inside your uterus, so that a radio frequency energy can burn the lining.

One moment the lining of my uterus was there, pink and smooth, the next it was white and flaky after she removed the ablation instrument wand. Then she placed the other stent in my tube with ease. The whole procedure only took about 30 minutes. When the nurse took out my IV, I realized that I must have had slight amnesia because I didn't remember having extra blankets placed on me because I had been shivering.

I was given a ginger soda and a package of crackers and could recover for as long as I wanted. My partner came in and took me to the front where I paid. I was coherent, able to walk on my own, just a little sweaty, and thousands of dollars poorer when I left the clinic.

I took my prescription of anti-nausea pills, painkiller tablets, and antibiotic capsules that I would have to take for the next two weeks to make sure that nothing got infected. For the next month I would have to have a panty liner to catch all the yellow ooze from the healing wound inside of me and wouldn't be able to have sex or sit in water.

After another long month, I was free. No more pain and no more blood. What was I going to do not having to feel so much pain and exhaustion? I began living life to the fullest. I didn't have to worry about planning events around my period. More importantly I could hold down a job, and have creative freedom without a period breaking my concentration. I know that some people would argue that having a period is "normal," but just because something is "normal" doesn't mean it's good. Is it good to hate yourself and not be happy because of your un-fulfilling life?

This procedure was right for me, but everyone will have to make that decision on your own. It was my last resort, and I'm glad I had it.

It's been two years since my ablation/Essure, and I haven't had any periods, painful uterine cramps, or pregnancies whatsoever. Sometimes I forget that I'm "supposed" to have periods, then I remember that day, and how happy I was to be saved.

DIGESTION SHIT

Wendy RM

It finally happened. Eighteen hours before stepping onto a plane, while walking to the bus stop for a final visit to one of my partners, I shit my pants.

Small stepped and thighs tensed, I hobbled the two long blocks back to my apartment, hoping against hope that I'd have the elevator to myself. When I got inside, I threw my bag down and told the cat sternly "Get out of the way. Don't touch me."

And now I'm sitting here, on the toilet, waiting again for mercy to visit my guts. I'm sitting scared that I won't be able to leave my home, scared to reach out to my partner and cancel. I don't want to concede to my sentence of sitting here. I don't want to cement my being stuck at home by texting "I might not make it."

While sitting and resisting this decision I feverishly scrape my nails into the mosquito bites I collected this weekend. I'm pleased by the simple satisfaction of scratching something that itches. The clear relationship between discomfort and relief is calming, even if the motivation itself is toxic. It's good to feel I have control over some things.

The bites I've been scratching are bleeding now. It's been ten full minutes since anything else has come out of me. Am I safe now? I think. I can hear the apartment manager vacuuming out in the hallway & for a moment I toil over whether or not I locked the front door. Part of me is convinced that she's going to come in and find me here like this. Half-naked and bent-double in the struggle of shitting. For a split second I fear that I will be evicted for my shits.

I snap to and recognize the absurdity of these fears.

Suddenly it occurs to me that I haven't eaten in eighteen hours. I feel hungry for the first time all morning (its almost one). Optimistically I take this as a sign that it's time to try putting pants on again.

Awkwardly, I rise and sit a few times to ensure that shifting doesn't dislodge any additional shit. I rise a final time and wipe. I pick up my soiled underwear and toss them into the garbage, sealing the top of the trash bag. I wash up meticulously and place bandages on my bleeding mosquito bites, my hunger slowly growing all the while.

When you have chronic digestive issues (and reliable food supply) the feeling of robust hunger can be such a gift. It tells me that my organs are working the way they were designed. I am personally grateful when I can feel my body aware of the nutrients it needs. This information tells me how to get closer to being healthy, a process that is never done.

.   .   .

I've left the apartment and taken the garbage out. On the top steps of the stairwell to the underground bus terminal I get a call. It's my partner asking where I am.

"I'm on my way. I got sick. It's been a rough morning."

I pause.

"Can we keep sex off the table for our date today? I'll tell you more when I get there."

I'm surprised at the strength and lack of fear in my voice. I feel completely willing, ready to tell him everything.

I take my seat on the bus, put on my headphones and pull from my bag the comforting snack of walnuts: perfect response to my joyously growling hunger. As I munch their delicious buttery meat, I feel strangely grateful. I'm relieved that now that it's happened, I know I'm capable of making it through at least this one thing I have feared so intensely.

Shitting my pants was bad, but certainly not as horrific and insurmountable an ordeal as I'd feared. I didn't become the disgusting disposable joke that "humorous" representations of diarrhea had lead me to believe I'd become. Instead, I realized that I have tools and I have rituals developed from previous negotiations with my bowel movements. Just as importantly, I have understanding loved ones who support me through my sickness and are patient with me when I can't always do the things we want to do together.

.   .   .

When it comes to my health, many things run counter to my wants. I have IBS and Generalized Anxiety Disorder. I must maintain both conditions attentively otherwise they feed into each other and leave me in a catch-22 of bad feelings. Sometimes I'm too nervous to eat. If I don't get enough nutrients my anxious tendencies intensify. And I forget to eat. Sometimes I can't eat at all.

My vague double diagnosis represents both the infuriating variety of my symptoms (physical and otherwise) and my inability to deeply explore the specifics of my health with a doctor. I'm uninsured. Since losing my health insurance last year I've been struggling to find ways of coping with the fear and discomfort in my life.

When I can manage it, writing about my experiences and sharing those words can help a lot. Your willingness to read these words goes a long way.

There're still parts of me that scream "Don't write about this! Girls don't talk about their shit! People will think you're doing femininity all wrong (never mind that I don't always consider myself a girl/feminine). People will think you're gross. They will be disgusted!" Or paradoxically even "You're such a fraud! You're just dredging this up to sound dramatic and get people to be interested in you. Stop throwing such a pity party."

Turns out the fear these self-suppressing voices drum up is far worse and certainly much shittier than the actual emergencies I've made it through.

The self-care skills I've developed combined with my stellar support network encourage me to fight back against these voices. If all goes well I find myself able to say, "Screw you fear. You ain't shit."

SERVICE DOG
Joe Biel

I've been living with Auto-immune (ANA) problems since I was about fifteen years old. ANA causes white blood cells, instead of fighting disease, infection, or foreign invaders, to attack my healthy body. Most weeks I spend at least one or two full days effectively in bed, either too tired or in too much pain to move. The pain is bad enough that it causes exhaustion and if I try to work through the pain, it just makes the following day even worse.

It took nearly twenty years of misdiagnosis and focusing on the wrong parts of my endocrine system before a doctor realized what was going on, why I hadn't been getting nutrients for so long, and how much damage had been done to my brain, body, and digestive system over time. It took a few more years and another doctor to figure out that the bacterial colony that's been ruling my body for the last few years originates from my small intestine rather than my colon, as previously thought. Despite the fact that there is no surgery, transplant, or even any lasting solution to get rid of Small Intestinal Bacterial Overgrowth (SIBO), it's comforting to know why I still feel terrible some days, even when I do everything as I'm supposed to.

Beyond medication, I largely control my problems through my diet. Avoiding foods that feed bacteria like sugar and simple carbs and focusing on fatty foods and greens. But still things go wrong sometimes.

One major problem that still plagues me is that my blood sugar is highly volatile. When the body doesn't have as much glucose as it needs, it begins cutting out non-mandatory functions. Eventually your glands will make the body pass out so it can maintain its vitals. My blood sugar drops can be unpredictable as well as sudden. For this reason it's generally not safe for me to go out after 7 PM. I've only had one bad fall in the last few years, cracking my head on concrete, but it was enough to change my habits.

But after all these years, the first positive: This disease allows me to qualify for an alert detection service dog who can go everywhere with me from the supermarket to Amtrak to restaurants to the thrift store.

A pre-requisite for getting a service dog in most states is having a medical condition that a dog can assist with. On top of that, a dog must be service-trained to be well-behaved in public places. A service dog is essentially invisible in private establishments and can't be refused as long as it well-behaved. Some people spend many hours training their own service dogs but most hire a professional trainer or even board a dog with the trainers. Most dogs that are domestic pets aren't able to be trained to do service work, or at least it would be incredibly difficult to train them from a patient owner. Normally a dog is selected for having general motivation and aptitude from a young age.

It took a few years to find a suitable and affordable dog trainer (the going rate is around $15,000) and then about six months to find a suitable dog that wasn't bred in some crazy situation to genetically be suited for this work. That stuff scared me and felt unethical.

I adopted Ruby on Valentine's Day, 2013, which seems appropriate. Since then we've had fabulous times. She sits in the bag on the front of my bike so she can look at me while we ride. She rests under my desk at work most of the day but pays attention all the time, in ways that really surprise and charm me.

Once I was watching a movie in bed because I was having ANA reactions and not feeling well. Ruby was curled up between my arm and my torso, tucked in as she's become quite adept at. Her training is to specifically be aware of changes inside my body that are communicated by different odors in my sweat, that would be undetectable to humans but can serve as early warning signs of something going wrong before medical equipment could detect it. In this particular case, even though she was soundly snoring, she was apparently still aware, because during a sad part in the movie, before I even began to cry, she was awake, alert, and comforting me. And it was comforting. Because I knew that she would be there in times when I needed her much more than this.

But then unexpected things started to happen. Crust punks would come up to me once per week and ask if my dog was really a service dog and how they could get a service dog. I understand why they would want to bring their dogs into places with them but it's not really an apples to apples situation. My dog serves a function in my life to increase my mobility and improves my quality of life that no other medical device could. And filling the city up with fake service dogs jeopardizes that.

Perhaps once per month when we are at a restaurant or public place, people will ask questions about the dog and her job. Legally, they can't ask any questions about my health or problems, and unless it's a friend, I don't feel like it's their business anyway. But because I look like a relatively-healthy, relatively-young person, people often assume that I am the dog trainer rather than the patient. They ask if I'll miss the dog after it's trained. It's also frequently assumed that the dog is some kind of scam. Sometimes people are rude to me about her, even when she's perfectly invisible and well-behaved.

I normally tell people that the dog is a medical alert service dog and that is sufficient and all I should need to tell them. Sometimes people with legitimate service needs ask me about her, how to get one, how to get it trained. I spent half an hour on the concrete porch of the post office detailing for a woman how to get a service dog and the struggles we went through.

Once in line at the credit union, the man in front of me in full military dress saw her working vest and watched Ruby sniff and look around and assess her environment and a full five minutes later he exclaimed, "Wow, she really knows what's going on around her!" which is perhaps the first person I've talked to that I really feel like understood the dynamic, albeit in his own way. But so far the biggest roadblock has been the confusion and misinformation about what service dogs are and what they do.

Maybe it's the piece of mind or my improving health regimen but I haven't had a major accident or injury since I adopted Ruby. She comes out with me if I need something from the store after 7 and while I often feel woozy and dizzy, knowing that she's there when a person couldn't be is often enough to increase my confidence.

Ruby and I continue to have our adventures. She forgets what her job is sometimes and then it becomes my job to positively reinforce her and give her enough love that we can remain as a functional team for years to come.

VEGANISM AND DIET
Natalie Taber

Sick, sick, sick all the time...I was in the hospital and out. I can't breathe. Phlegm. Fevers. Coughing. Lots of reading alone. Hot, cold, skinny, fragile. I was ten years old, 5' 1" and 73 lbs. Then a lifetime of bronchitis, strep throat, and tonsillitis.

I grew up poor in the Arkansas Ozarks and received a first-hand introduction to the factory farming industry. I became a politically-motivated vegan activist at 15 years old. My bronchitis and respiratory problems disappeared for five years.

But after seven years of a strict vegan diet, major cognitive problems were apparent. The soy and wheat didn't feel right in my body. I was showing clear signs of having an auto-immune disease. I was having regular panic attacks that had the odd mental content of seafood. I felt mood swings that I hadn't before—emotional and mental instability of a new variety.

I tried everything to help my body while remaining true to my ideal. I read, researched, and worked with a vegan dietitian. It was hard to let go of the politics and listen to my body. It was hard to let go of the righteousness and listen to my mind. I was hurting. It wasn't working and I knew it. But I told myself that I should be able to follow this diet, that I should be able to live to these ethics, values, and, politics. Forever.

It was right. I should be able to do this...why wasn't it working?

But the body can only take so much abuse and deprivation, even in the name of "health", even in the name of "right." I wasn't listening to my body. Instead I was listening to "experts"—doctors, activists, and philosophers who said that it was a doable and healthy way to live. I was trying to force my body to conform to rules that it was clearly rejecting.

It took being laid flat out and given the choice of narcotics (for debilitating migraines while vegan and pregnant) or trying to change my diet that led to ending twelve years of veganism. The change that had resolved one set of serious health problems had created another.

Veganism had a lot of positives for me—it healed my body from serious health problems; it brought my daily practice closer to my ideals; and it severed most of my ties to mainstream food culture.

It's been seven years since I began eating animal foods. I began by eating local goat dairy. The first meat I ate came from a farm down the road from Daefflers Quality Meats, an ultra-local butcher shop. I suffered no ill effects, only positives. I still stay away from conventionally grown, raised, or processed foods—animal and plant alike. In these seven years, my health has drastically improved. I'm hardly ever sick, my cognitive functions have returned to normal, the mood swings are gone, the panic attacks where I only think of seafood are gone. My health isn't perfect, but it is more balanced. When it starts to get out of balance, I search for what will return me closer to balance. It involves a little wu—asking my body what would help, listening, and trying it out. It usually works.

I think the biggest problem with how I was raised, in terms of my health, was the enforcement, by my mom and my culture, of the strict notion that someone else knew what was good for me and my body. If I was sick all the time, it signified a weakness with my body, with me. It took until I was an adult to realize that it was the dairy that had made me ill; not a failing on my part.

But I failed the same way a second time when I thought there was, again, something wrong with me that I couldn't stay vegan and be healthy. As a culture we have an unhealthy focus on the short term. It's worth expanding on instant gratification in the context of our health. Listening to your body, especially when you aren't used to doing so, requires a longer term. It requires flexibility. Even if something works for a year, it doesn't mean it will work for you always, or that it will work for anyone else ever.

If you are having major respiratory problems, eczema, or urinary tract infections, completely cut out cow dairy for a month. The difficulty in changing your lifestyle will be worth the positive results. Goat dairy is still an option if you are having trouble.

Without a question, being irresponsible for ourselves is the most unhealthy thing in our culture that is still treated as acceptable. With the birth of my second child, I had an amazing midwife who had a condition for only accepting clients that they were responsible for themselves; who didn't look for salvation from the outside—from a doctor, hospital, midwife, partner, or anyone else. There is a big difference between being "independent" and being responsible for yourself. You can depend on a doctor, partner, midwife or anyone in a healthy way. The problem occurs when you expect that anyone else is ultimately responsible for your choices and your outcomes.

My culture encourages my health through fermentation fervor, priobiotics, and being as close to our food as possible. One of the most important things in my culture is the support and encouragement of informed critical thinking. Truth is not a commodity that doesn't belong to any particular government, philosophy, religion, socio-econoic class, product, or xyz-industrial complex. My culture has supported me doing reasoned, purposeful, and politically challenging things that are different from what is found acceptable in mainstream culture.

Health has many dimensions—physical, emotional, and psychological—and, in some ways, I've only dealt here with the physical side of things. It is important to note that I had to overcome serious psychological and emotional barriers as well, but that's its own story. So let's just say I feel the happiest and healthiest when people trust me and value my words and intuitions.

LET ME TALK ABOUT FEELINGS

Xena Goldman

For as long as I can remember, I've been an emotional chick; not in a Let's-Go-See-A-Rom-Com-Tonight, kind of way, but in a I-Can't-Stop-Crying-For-Absolutely-No-Reason kind of way. Growing up, I remember the confusion of being inexplicably cheerless, or moved to tears by a poignant McDonald's commercial. I knew what "suicide" meant before I learned what sex was. By the time I finished Middle School, I had seen dozens of therapists, yet felt no better off as a result.

In my teens, my previously stellar grades began to plummet, as I recognized it was easier to convince myself I didn't care than to try to explain to anybody that I was having panic attacks; something I didn't know was a real thing for many years. I felt horribly misunderstood, and fell into a punk/stoner/rebel crowd, which turned stylish brooding into an Olympic sport. Instead of treating depression, my peers looked for ways to cultivate it, channel it into art, music, and amateur philosophical reflection. We shoved towels under our door so our parents wouldn't smell the weed, and would sit for hours in a haze of smoke and Jim Morison's drug-induced musings. Nothing ever got solved, except finding ways to pass the time.

After high school, I moved from Chicago to Minneapolis, where I left behind my friends to start anew. Minnesota winters and the menacing time-management monster of college skyrocketed my depression and anxiety. Finally, I turned to prescription medication for help.

For those of you who don't know, going on a quest for a medication match is like joining a dating website: for months you flirt with the idea of a future with your new find, to later discover a slew of chemical byproducts, packed haphazardly in the baggage they slowly sneak into your apartment. Nausea, blurred vision, extreme drowsiness and intense mood swings were just a few of the knickknacks I found wedged in the sock drawer of my limbic system. Relationships, grades, and self-esteem took blow after blow as I tried to make peace with the orgy of substances repositioning themselves in my body. Libido disappearing acts were corrected by additional pills. Side effects were swept under the rug of new prescriptions and new side effects.

I've been called "weak" by so-called friends who believed I was using pills as an easy way out. I filled out Academic Disability paperwork, as though I didn't feel handicapped enough without legal paperwork to confirm it. I've tried St. John's Wort, light therapy, meditation, and liquor. I've let boyfriends treat me badly because it beat the abuse I'd inflict on myself in solitude. I've felt utterly alone, useless. I've gotten to lows so low that I've wanted to die. And then, somehow, I found myself wanting to live again.

Medication bartenders aren't always spot on, and even now I sometimes wonder if my pills make me more shaken than stirred. They don't work for everyone, but for me, in the end, they've proved to be more helpful than hurtful. Still, pills aren't the Be All End All. Though they can be a valuable tool to keep calm, being healthy is so much more than just that; just like taking aspirin won't make your headache go away if you don't turn the death metal off.

The period of learning what makes you healthy can be one of the most isolating experiences that a person can go through, but also one of the most rewarding. For me, it means cutting out heavy drinking (because my meds and booze don't mix well), not staying out late so I can wake up early to go running (releasing endorphins is a huge help), not slamming coffee like a 1950s beatnik (too much caffeine is bad for my nerves), and surrounding myself with positive-minded people. Our bad habits are often our only friends, but staying healthy means learning when it's time to see other people.

Also, giving in to immediate impulses, like going out to a movie when I know I have things to do, tends to lead to more lasting feelings of guilt and remorse. Time management and putting weight on the things that are truly important allow me to throw away the invitation to the Self Hate party before I can even think about RSVPing. As corny as it sounds, good health—whether physical or mental—stems from self love. That translates to treating yourself like a friend, and not beating yourself up when you behave in a way that you're not proud of.

Our culture may never fully accept the legitimacy of mental health problems: I've been denied by multiple health insurance companies that don't want to provide care to me, and rejected by men who refuse to date someone who would take prescription medication. Still, I'm not about to shy away from talking about the matter just because it makes people uncomfortable. It takes courage and strength to talk about that which scares us and about the obstacles that we overcome. Now, if anyone calls me weak, I assume they are ignorant or have their own demons that they haven't been able to break up with yet. My emotions are a part of me, and despite all the grief they've caused me, I wouldn't trade them for the world.

WHO CAN YOU TRUST?

Robert Earl Sutter III

....

I was beaten and tormented all through grade school. People that I called my friends would hold my arms and punch me in the stomach until I couldn't breathe. I tried to smuggle a weapon to school to defend myself, a dull butter knife, but it fell out of my coat when my mom dropped me off. She yelled at me and I got in trouble. I couldn't even articulate in words how bad the bullies were. How was she supposed to know?

After my family moved to Alaska, the beatings and torment continued at a different elementary school until I snapped and went violently psychotic on another kid. My teacher dragged me to the office where, tragically, the principal decided the appropriate punishment would be to beat my ass with a wooden paddle and put me in solitary confinement for a few weeks, as if it was some sort of prison.

Then when I graduated and was thrown in with the big kids in high school, I was again beaten and tormented. It was here where the most brutal attack happened to me. Riding the bus to my friend's house one afternoon a bully told me he was going to kick my ass when I got off the bus. I wasn't afraid. I was with friends. I got off with my friends and was hit in the back of the head. My glasses flew off and I was nearly blind. The bully knocked me down and jumped on top of me, punching me in the face until blood spurted out. I spotted a metal fence post on the ground next to me. I reached for it, a weapon to defend myself, but it was out of reach. The bully saw me try to grab for it and it made him even crazier. I really thought he was going to kill me. The bus driver did nothing even as it unfolded right in front of the bus. My "friends" watched while he beat me. They did nothing, afraid of being beaten themselves.

Every time I went to school after that brutal attack at the bus stop I wondered if I would be beaten again. Sometimes I would see the bully and he would mock me, surrounded by his gang of friends. Laughing at me, taunting me. I will probably not feel comfortable seeing groups of two or more men looking my way until I die. Unless it's in a queer space; that feels different to me.

For years the torment and beatings continued until my immediate family were the only ones left in my circle of trust. To this day, the slightest betrayal against me is subject to total dismissal of friendship. You only get one chance and then you are out. I won't even talk about the events that eroded my trust, because confrontation could equal being beaten. If not physically then a psychic, emotional beating. That's the haggard child that still exists in my adult body, in my mind, my emotions. I have to pay serious attention to it, because even those survival mechanisms aren't working for me in adult life, they just make me feel lonely and look crazy and scary just like the bullies who did this to me.

Damn those boys. What wretched abuse they must have suffered in their lives to have such brutal hate bottled up in them.

The fact that my friends stood and watched was very meaningful to me. Since nobody of any gender came to my rescue, nobody of any race or age or class helped me, it taught me that I could not trust anyone at all. I'm now 42 years old and there are few people in the world that I trust. Often I find myself alone, by choice. Probably as a result of these very circumstances, people evoke anger and fear in me, to the point where I avoid them to protect myself. It is difficult to cultivate friendships. Many years of public schooling taught me that other people are not to be trusted. You can't even trust your friends because they will fucking watch you get beaten. That's what the traumatic experiences of my youth taught me, over and over again. Since the only person I could trust was myself, I sought myself out, and found spaces where only I existed, and those were the spaces I felt safe and I cherished those spaces. Out behind the portable buildings, down by the creek, in the forest, behind the bushes, in my room at home, in my car, somewhere in a café with my back to the wall and headphones on so I can't hear the vicious things that might come out of people's mouths.

This is what is called Post Traumatic Stress Disorder. Several people recommended I get Eye Movement Desensitization & Reprocessing therapy, or EMDR, which deals with processing traumatic memories and reprograms your brain to use healthier coping mechanisms. Sounds good.

I could have been a school shooter, but I never had access to guns. I guess I made it through that potential fate. So here I am and fucked up. Surviving. Dealing with the result of another family's generational violence that has been passed down and outwards for who knows how long. Trying to end it here, now, tonight.

Recognizing that something is wrong is the first step towards being healthy.

COMING OUT TRANSGENDERED

Allison Ryder

Having lost my job as a mortician due to being a part-time transgender (full time since the day I was fired) woman, I had to retrain and went to phlebotomy class. Getting my name and gender changed legally required that I have a paper signed by my doctor stating that I *am* a transgender woman. This was the first time my doctor had met me as Allison. It was nerve-wracking but he was cool with it, even saying that 'he' felt bad that he couldn't tell "something was up" with me sooner. I had only seen him as a patient five or six times and, as I told him, I had a lot of practice "hiding." The clinic even had, on their admission sheet: M, F, TG so I marked F and TG.

If another transgender person needed a doctor, I would recommend my doctor and/or the Hillside Clinic on Laws Avenue in Ukiah.

Eat good food, *tell* yourself to be healthy (hey, I *want* to live, right? I *want* to live as long as I can as the woman I AM), think healthy and stay mentally healthy.

Allowing yourself to be dragged down by depression, eating shitty food, not believing in yourself. Those are very important to one's health.

Being depressed. Falling · into the pit of depression and...'accepting' that that is normal. Stay off drugs and away from crap people who will not improve your life.

Reading about and meeting other transgender people. Not feeling like I'm the only one in the world who is like me. There are other transgender girls and I enjoy having met them and associating with them via the internet.

How I was raised had nothing to do with me being transgender, even so, my mother did her best to raise us right. We had food (though maybe not the best) and she cares about us (my sisters and I). She 'accepts' me as Alli even though she is reluctant to meet me as her daughter.

Knowing that I am a good person, knowing that I am not the only transgender person in the world, being accepted as a woman by my friends (many of whom knew me from before my transition) and knowing that I *will* make it gives me confidence that I survive in this world.

DENTAL BASICS

Dr. Elizabeth Meyer, D.D.S.

....

I have been practicing general dentistry in a small farming town in the middle of Ohio for 12 1/2 years. I like my job a lot and am still fascinated by dental curiosities on a daily basis. I enjoy fixing mouths, whether the fix involves a small filling, cosmetic bonding, braces, or a full mouth extraction with a shiny new set of dentures. One of my favorite aspects of being a dentist is the education of the souls who find their way into my super-comfy chairs. I never get tired of answering questions and doling out advice, even when it seems like no one is listening. But you'll listen, won't you?

The Basics

Everyone should brush their teeth *at least* twice a day. Seriously, you should always brush your teeth at least twice per day. It doesn't matter if your brush costs 25 cents or $100, as long as you spend 1-2 minutes with the bristles against your teeth and you cover all surfaces of every tooth. In my opinion, a soft brush is best because it is flexible enough to reach between teeth and doesn't have a tendency to damage your gums like a hard-bristled brush can. I like to use a toothpaste containing fluoride once a day for its decay-fighting abilities (I've read enough long-term studies to believe that it's a good thing). If you're feeling ambitious, learn to floss properly and take 2 minutes to do it daily, or at least a couple times a week. When you eat sweets, highly acidic foods, sticky carbs like bread or chips, or even corn on the cob, brush or at least rinse your mouth with water. Use a mouthwash if you'd like, it won't hurt anything.

Visiting the Dentist

Some dentists are cocky and mean. Some hygienists inflict pain when they clean your teeth. You need to find an office where they make you feel mentally and physically comfortable. If you can't, you will hate going to the dentist. Not all procedures are pleasant, but dental work never has to hurt. There's almost always a way to make it better. Ask if you feel like you want to try laughing gas, need to be more numb, want them to put numbing cream on you gums to clean your teeth or if you don't like the way something looks or how your bite feels. A good dentist wants to know what will make you happier.

A dentist or hygienist will suggest you have bitewing x-rays taken annually. Sometimes, an x-ray is the only way to find decay between your teeth until the cavity gets very large or deep, then you may need a root canal or extraction. We also like to see people twice a year for a cleaning and an exam. This way, we can catch problems early, answer questions, and prevent deep tartar and plaque build from becoming too heavy. If you can't see a dentist regularly, at least try to have an exam and x-rays every few years and practice great hygiene at home.

If you dislike having your teeth worked on, the worst thing you can do is squirm, complain and refuse to open wide. That pisses off the staff, makes a procedure take a *lot* longer and we will bitch about you later. Just open wide and try to cooperate.

Dental Care for Kids

As soon as a baby sprouts a tooth, it needs to be cleaned. Brush it, wipe it with a cloth, rub it with a clean finger, whatever. Never let a baby or toddler go to bed with a bottle or sippy-cup of juice, milk or anything except water. Baby-bottle tooth decay (this applies to cups too) is sad. A three year old kid who has to have four top front teeth pulled and eight molars capped has been abused, and I've seen it many times. Please take care of your little ones' teeth how you should take care of your own, and treat their precious bodies like little temples when deciding what they eat and drink. They deserve a good start. Once a toddler can spit, I recommend using a children's toothpaste with a small amount of fluoride.

In Summary

I must now reiterate the need to brush your teeth. I won't drink water, eat breakfast or kiss my husband and kids in the morning until my teeth are brushed and my mouth doesn't taste like bacteria stew. At bedtime, even if I'm exhausted, have the flu, have been drinking or I'm nauseous with all-day morning sickness, I brush my teeth—365 days a year. I put a toothbrush in my mouth before I read or rock my kids to sleep and curl up in bed. The best way to avoid huge dental expenses and lots of potential problems is to be proactive and practice prevention. Let a dentist help you keep your mouth healthy, but you can do the majority of the work yourself!

And Finally

Don't let the fact that your parents, grandparents or siblings have awful teeth convince you that you should have problems. Nor will you lose a tooth for every child you bear. My folks both had dentures in their 20s. I've had 3 kids and have lost no teeth other than my whizzies and am capable of maintaining good oral health. *Very* few dental problems are genetic and 99.97% of them are due to poor oral hygiene and a lousy diet. Be accountable!

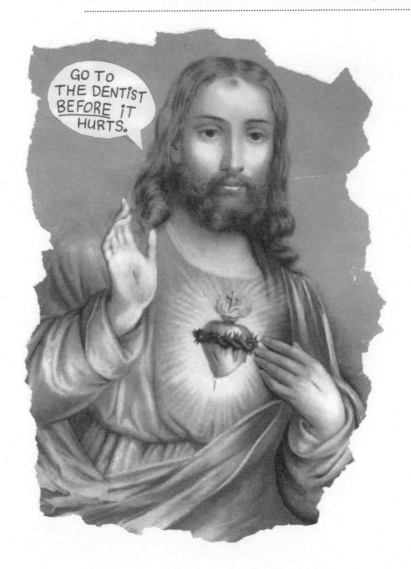

QUITTING SMOKING
Robert Earl Sutter III

It was a long and lonely winter on the lower slopes of the White Mountain. At last the snow had melted. Spring was on, the time had come. May 8th: I stop smoking corporate tobacco products. I would like to thank and apologize to my friends who were around me at that time. It seems strange now that I ever smoked.

I used to get out of bed and bike through the freezing night to purchase the stuff. When I was broke I rode my bike to the hospital because there would always be half smoked cigarettes in the ashtrays outside, or walk around the neighborhood staring at the ground, hunting for a gutter snipe. I remember being hungry and spending my very last dollars on smokes instead of food.

How did I get out?

I started smoking when I was 21 and stopped when I was 39. Nicotine is one of the most addictive substances on Earth. Most people start when they are teenagers but I was fortunate that my parents didn't smoke, so I didn't have it around to tempt me, the easy access. I stopped and started a few times, but what finally locked quitting down for me was doing the research on what Nicotine does to your brain, how it creates a lie of satisfaction, in the same way that corporate advertisements create a false sense of happiness in us.

Corporate tobacco could be the ultimate insidious product, because it physically enslaves the mind through chemical reactions. The realization that being a smoker did not make me any kind of rebel but a tool of corporate profit changed my attitude. By purchasing cigarettes I wasn't living the high life. I was altering the chemical makeup of my brain to increase the profits of corporations. Oh yeah, and damaging my throat, lungs, heart, and body.

I still have some addictions too: sugar; caffeine. It's more serious than it seems. I've been stealing cookies, and when I overdose on caffeine I'll be riding my bike and flip off every car that comes near me. I'm working on that.

a craving for nicotine will last no longer than 3 minutes. Time it.

Nicotine is an insecticide used to keep insects off the tobacco plant's leaves. Nicotine is also nearly chemically identical to a neurotransmitter in the brain that controls the flow of Dopamine, the brain's Motivation Neurotransmitter. The Dopamine circuits of the brain teach us important lessons using a powerful wanting sensation. When we feel hunger, our Dopamine circuits are being stimulated, and when it is satisfied, the body stops the dopamine flow. The brain then records exactly how this satisfaction was achieved and hard wires Dopamine neuro-transmission circuits into our conscious memory. Nicotine hijacks this system, causes Dopamine to be released, and manufactures the desire to smoke tobacco. It's a total lie, a chemical scam. By smoking tobacco you aren't giving your body something it needs, you're giving it something it's been told to want by the injection of an outside chemical.

But everyone's body is different and ten percent of people are actually immune to becoming addicted to Nicotine.

But smoking makes you feel good, right? Do you remember what it was like before you smoked? Did you feel good then? Can you remember?

Nicotine is a stimulant, activating the body's fight or flight response and giving a brief high which becomes part of the Dopamine circuit memory. These vivid memories replace life before Nicotine. Now with the brain reprogrammed by Nicotine. Who do you believe, your brain that tells you to smoke tobacco, or the outside world that tells you to stop? Smoking tobacco will kill 5 million people this year. People who smoke will die 14 years earlier than people who don't. Such facts will not make you quit.

The only thing that can overcome Nicotine's chemical programming in your brain is your conscious mind. If you become educated and aware of what Nicotine is doing to your brain, you can decide to be free. If you understand that your brain has a permanent disorder activated by Nicotine, you can make the decision to never inhale corporate tobacco again.

When I quit, I tapered off, down to one cigarette in the morning and one at night. I dont think this had any effect on the chemical situation in my brain, but after several weeks it reduced the amount of time I was physically smoking, breaking me from the habit, and pushing me to put other things in my hands, preparing me to quit.

Navigating the symptoms of withdrawal is not easy. The first three days are challenging and full of irrational emotional outbursts, anger

if you can make it thru 3 days of not smoking, the worst cravings are over.

and hate. Take a few days off, take a week vacation if you can! Avoid stress. Avoid situations that are smoking cues. Hang out with your trusted support person. After about ten days things get wildly better. After several months you notice incredible changes. The constant flow of energy makes you feel like a superhero and the even flow of emotion feels great.

Instead of feeling bad and then smoking to feel good, I feel good all the time, like a smooth criminal!

Essential Facts for Quitting:

Nicotine dependency is a mental illness.

There is no cure, the mental illness is permanent. Years of Nicotine use have left us wired for relapse. One single puff of tobacco re-activates all the receptors, take just one puff, and you will be re-captured.

Certain situations will trigger Nicotine use such as being at a party, a live music show, on lunch break, after eating a meal. Specific times, places, people.

Further reading:
www.whyquit.com
http://www.cdc.gov/tobacco

ABUSIVE RELATIONSHIPS

Dominick Brooks

Though there's no way to know for sure, I think both of my parents had Asperger's Syndrome. My dad was calm and polite throughout his whole life but his jokes were very obtuse. He preferred to be alone and he would often state the opposite of the obvious without any expression. If it was raining, he'd say, "Great weather today." He seemed to naturally have the skills of an engineer and a complete understanding of all things mechanical. As a kid I thought he knew everything but he could hold me in his lap and I could feel absolutely nothing. While he was a bit socially cold, he was a nice person, when he remembered to try.

My mom, on the other hand, also had clear Aspie symptoms but her personality manifested her asocial nature differently. She was emotionally dead but knew how to use emotions to get what she wanted. You had to speak in clear words that couldn't be misunderstood. She had emotions, of course, but mostly anger and frustration. She was also highly manipulative and would knowingly lie to us to get what she wanted.

It's said that the two kinds of people who date aspies are other aspies and people with bad boundaries, who don't walk away when their communication is lost and their feelings are repeatedly hurt. My parents were no exception and perhaps reflected both kinds of relationships.

From the time I was very young, I remember my mom being repeatedly physically violent towards my dad, my sister, and me. She would lose her temper, beat us, and then blame us for the beating, saying that we had "caused" it. Now, when it's spelled out this way, it sounds ridiculous; but when you're six years old and the only person who has ever shown you any emotional warmth or responsiveness tells you that it was your fault that you were beaten and shamed, you tend to believe it and do everything you can to get back into their good graces. I remember sitting for hours next to my mom, while she watched television, nervously clutching my security blanket after a prolonged beating. She would anxiously pick at her nails until they were bloody. To this day, the sounds of someone picking their nails or scraping a metal spoon against a metal pot give me triggering shivers and can cause me to physically recoil. I'm not sure if I associate them with the pain and fear of my childhood or the regret of trying to get back into the good graces of someone who was incapable of loving me the way I needed to be loved.

Needless to say, all of this did not do much to prepare me for adulthood or to shape good boundaries for myself. I continued routine contact with my parents after I moved out. When my dad died it seemed to make my mom and I closer for a brief period but it was likely just one of her deceptions. She had always insisted to me, in confidence, that everything that went wrong when I was a child was his fault.

I had been in serious romantic relationships throughout my teens, but my lack of boundaries and my own emotional retardation had always given pause to my dates, eventually scaring them away. When I turned 20 I got into a different kind of serious relationship, that felt different, though I couldn't put my finger on it at the time.

We would argue for hours, just shouting back and forth. I was frequently shamed, sometimes publicly, often in front of my friends. I was called all kinds of names and insults, from stupid to lazy to boring to useless. Everyday. I didn't know how to do the dishes right. I didn't say the right thing. Every argument or situation was my fault, even if we both played a role. It eroded what self-esteem I had left. I didn't have the confidence or awareness to leave. I didn't recognize the dynamics at play. In many ways it was comforting because it reminded me of my relationship with my mother growing up.

Two years later we got married. I thought all relationships were like this as it was the only kind I had ever known. I felt afraid and horrible all the time. I walked around my life on eggshells and went out of my way to get out of the house and spend time with friends. I can't imagine my partner was happy either. My ex-partner lacked the boundaries to advocate for themself and name what the problems were in our situation, so instead they lashed out. At me. We were together for another two years before calling it quits, and even then neither of us had the solid boundaries to properly break off our lives from each other, even though it clearly made everyone around the situation miserable.

I spent the next four years in therapy. We delved through my family past and I recognized signs of abuse as far back as I could remember with my grandfather. In the final year of therapy I was given the Asperger's test and scored a 98%. I had always joked about having Asperger's Syndrome after I learned about its existence, but I was too old to have been tested for it as a child and I have no children, so it was not discovered sooner.

But it put my life in perspective and helped me move on from my childhood and my twenties. And while I don't want my mom to be a part of my life and I will always carry many years of horrifying memories, of watching her beat my dad to a pulp and worse, I learned to understand what she was going through and eventually forgive her. The emotions she was engaging with was a result of society not having the answers that she needed, to unravel her intense feelings and how the world was not designed in a way that worked for her.

While I'm sure I was quite a handful to deal with, I have a harder time forgiving my ex for engaging in a power struggle and using all of my needs as a way to hold power over me, and then telling me it was my fault. Strangely, I found that violence, while painful and scary, was not nearly as scary as the kind of control manifested through threats, fear, and utter manipulation of my emotions.

A decade later I'm in a good place, with a good handle on my Asperger's, and in a healthy relationship for the last five years. We have excellent communication, a lot of love, and can work through our needs mutually. Like many people with Asperger's, I look at my younger self and I don't see myself. I see a person that looks as foreign as a stranger on the street, deep-seated scars notwithstanding.

I take it as my personal responsibility to end this cycle of abuse. Right here.

BUILDING THE WORLD
WE WANT TO SEE
Buck Angel

Over the years, I have felt tremendous vocal and emotional support from the trans community. The documentary film *Sexing the Transman* was a big hit with the trans male community. Many people wrote to tell me how excited they were that I was discussing this forbidden topic of men enjoying their trans bodies sexually. It felt necessary to bring a positive outlook to the world and to help other trans people do the same. The support I receive everyday is amazing. I know how hard it is to transition and have learned that being positive is the way to go and I know that so many others are having that same experience.

I'm proud to see the changes and awareness we've created over the last twenty years, but I'm equally concerned at the frequency with which I see members of my community feeling the need to tear down other trans people.

It seems that whenever a trans person achieves a certain level of success as an advocate, that rather than being supportive of someone who has a greater opportunity to raise rights and awareness about trans issues in the broader world, the responses are critical about every last detail of the person's approach.

Now, I understand that not every trans voice is representative of everyone and that there is a value for "calling people out on their shit" but tearing down our advocates, our activists, and our most vocal and powerful allies will only result in a lack of progress for trans rights, among other things. I don't shy away from being called out on my shit. I am not perfect and like to learn if I am doing something wrong. But doing it in a public forum is not the ideal way to do this.

I'm not saying not to be critical. But I'm asking you to look at the bigger picture, at the campaign, where the world is going, and how we can raise awareness and be more respected when we get there. When I did an interview for my new dating site, I talked about why it is so important to have sites like mine that help disclose that you are trans right out of the gate. Disclosure is important, among other reasons, because it eliminates the potential for any number of bad things that could happen. I used an example of a trans woman going on a date with a cis-gendered man. When the possibility of sex comes into play, if she has not disclosed that she is a trans person, there is the potential for her getting beaten up or even killed. Several responses publicly accused me of victim blaming, a very real phenomenon, that while, perhaps my words were unclear, I had no intention of expressing. I was hoping that, while everyone's experience is different, trans people would see disclosure as part of being proud of who you are.

But instead, the trans community beat me up for that. I suspect other people have seen similar behavior in other situations. I was called all kinds of names and cyber-bashed to hell. It's crushing when your own community—the community that theoretically relates to the way that you have suffered more than anyone else—is the one feeling the need to tear you down, doing so with abusive language. I've seen enough of that in the cold, uncaring world. I wished others could have given me the benefit of the doubt, or at least asked questions before mimicking the way that mainstream culture creates cycles of making each other feel terrible.

Political concerns aside, if the goal is to broaden awareness and shape a message, criticisms about someone's approach tend to work best as loving reminders about other struggles, about things they may have neglected, and about how things could be done better next time. Public campaigns attacking our own leaders tend to accomplish little beyond making us appear disorganized, sloppy, and like we just want to fight with each other about semantics.

It is important to understand that by publicly humiliating a trans person you are doing what our political and social opponents want to see. They want to see us defeated. They do not want us to be organized and strong. I am a big believer of the power in numbers. If our whole LGBTQ community learned to understand that we all have similar goals, like living a life free of hate, then we could rule the world.

Remember Harvey Milk, the first openly queer visionary to be elected to public office in 1978 in California? He brought all manner of queer struggles to a national spotlight and created an inspiring legacy for queer people for years to come. That's not to say that Harvey wasn't without his critics or that he didn't slip up from time to time. He was rejected by the existing queer political establishment when he showed up on the scene in San Francisco and many of his critics were slow to be won over, essentially telling him and his radical approach to wait their turn on the sidelines.

But the community eventually came to understand the importance of creating a social movement, ending police attacks on queer establishments, not accepting less than they wanted, and what was needed to project publicly: Building allies in unlikely places, and most importantly, projecting a united front. Harvey did all these things and is now remembered as a natural leader. Despite criticisms, he created a role that it's hard to think of a trans person occupying today.

In my future utopia, all kinds of trans people are respected and criticism is delivered to other people who have struggled similarly in ways that are supportive and build a movement, not slow one down.

So here's my proposal: We each work on being the best advocate that we can be and work to build a community rather than tearing each other down. And it's okay to tell people how they can do better, but it's probably more effective to do so with the loving tone that you would communicate to someone you care deeply about.

AN INADVERTENTLY COMPELLING ARGUMENT FOR NATIONAL HEALTH CARE IN FIVE MUTUALLY INCRIMINATING SCENES

Ayun Halliday

Scene One

HEARTY AUTOMATED WHITE MALE: Good morning! Thank you for calling Sunspire. If you are a health care provider, press pound now. For information on becoming a Sunspire Child Health Plus member, press pound three.

LESS HEARTY AUTOMATED SPANISH-SPEAKING FEMALE: *(translation of the above)*

HEARTY AUTOMATED WHITE MALE: Members, enter your identification number followed by the pound sign. Enter only the numbers. Skip any letters or symbols.

(The Conflict-Avoiding, Procrastination-Prone Artist Mother of Epileptic Child, otherwise known as OUR HEROINE, squints through an obsolete contact lens prescription at a plastic card she fishes from her battered wallet.)

HEARTY AUTOMATED WHITE MALE: Please hold while we check our eligibility records. *(Pause)* Enter the patient's date of birth as an eight digit number, month-month- day-day -year-year-year-year, followed by the pound sign.

(OUR HEROINE, one eye twitching involuntarily, does so.)

HEARTY AUTOMATED WHITE MALE: For claims, press one. Coverage, benefits, and premiums, two. Precertification, three. All other services and information, four.

(OUR HEROINE hesitates, before hastily stabbing one of the aforementioned numerals.)

Pause

FEMALE REPRESENTATIVE NUMBER 1: Good morning, thank you for calling Sunspire. My name is Mrs. Drrwsschkx. May I-

OUR HEROINE: Hi, yes, my daughter's got epilepsy and-

FEMALE REPRESENTATIVE NUMBER 1: May I have your name, Ma'am?

OUR HEROINE: Oh, uh, sure, my first name is A as in apple, y as in yellow, u as in umbrella, n as in Nancy. The last name's H-a-l-l-i-d-as-in-David-a-y, but my daughter's got her father's last name, which is K-as-in-kitten-o-t-i-s-as-in-Sam.

(Pause. Audible tapping on a computer keyboard.)

FEMALE REPRESENTATIVE NUMBER 1: Would that be Milo?

OUR HEROINE: No, India. Milo's her brother.

FEMALE REPRESENTATIVE NUMBER 1: India, huh? That's real unique.

OUR HEROINE: Oh, uh, thanks.

FEMALE REPRESENTATIVE NUMBER 1: Different. May I get India's date of birth?

OUR HEROINE, suppressing irritation at having to resupply this information, resupplies this information.

FEMALE REPRESENTATIVE NUMBER 1: Thank you, Mrs. Kotis. And Mrs. Kotis, can I get you to verify your home address for me?

(OUR HEROINE overlooks the surname error and states her home address. Pause. Then...)

FEMALE REPRESENTATIVE NUMBER 1: Thank you for calling Sunspire, Mrs. Kotis. How may I assist you today?

OUR HEROINE: Uh, well, my daughter has epilepsy and her seizures have been increasing so her doctor had us do an EK-, I mean, an EEG, and

we did it, except now I just got a bill from Sunspire for a thousand dollars, saying it wasn't covered.

FEMALE REPRESENTATIVE NUMBER 1: Can you give me the date the service was performed?

(OUR HEROINE'S hands shake as she supplies the date printed on a statement received two month's prior.)

FEMALE REPRESENTATIVE NUMBER 1: Thank you. Just one moment while my computer searches for ... okay, thank you for waiting. I'm seeing here that Dr. Neurospikowski is not one of our participating providers-

OUR HEROINE: Dr. Neurospin... I don't know who that is.

FEMALE REPRESENTATIVE NUMBER 1: He doesn't participate, so any services provided by him wouldn't be covered. To qualify for coverage, you'd have to see a participating provider.

OUR HEROINE: I don't know who that is, though....

FEMALE REPRESENTATIVE NUMBER 1: Our records show that this service was performed by Dr. Neurospikowsky.

OUR HEROINE: Yeah, except that can't be right because our neurologist's name is Dr. Head.

FEMALE REPRESENTATIVE NUMBER 1: This claim was submitted by a Dr. Neurospikowsky.

OUR HEROINE: Except how can that be? Our doctor's name is Dr. Head.

FEMALE REPRESENTATIVE NUMBER 1: Is he the one who performed the service?

OUR HEROINE: *(Uncertainly)* A technician performed the service. There wasn't any doctor.

FEMALE REPRESENTATIVE NUMBER 1: Then what I would suggest is call the doctor and ask him to resubmit the claim.

OUR HEROINE: *(defeated and submissive, wishing a good fairy would appear at the window to relieve her of this burden)* Oh…okay.

• • •

Scene Two
Many months, possibly as much as two years, later

The HEARTY AUTOMATED WHITE MALE and LESS HEARTY AUTOMATED SPANISH-SPEAKING FEMALE offer OUR HEROINE, the Conflict-Avoiding, Procrastination-Prone Artist Mother of the Epileptic Child their standard greetings. Allowing her mind to wander, she inadvertently selects the incorrect numeric prompt, and after some telephonic thrashing about, finds herself disconnected. Muttering venomously, she redials the number on the back of the epileptic child's membership card, and is subjected to identical automated greetings. Listening more actively, she succeeds in pushing all the requisite buttons. There follows an interminable ten minute interval, after which OUR HEROINE is patched through to FEMALE REPRESENTATIVE NUMBER 43

OUR HEROINE: Hi, my daughter's got epilepsy and-

FEMALE REPRESENTATIVE NUMBER 43: Can I get your name, Ma'am?

OUR HEROINE: A as in apple, y as in yellow, u as in umbrella, n as in Nancy, last name H-a-l-l-i-d-as-in-David-a-y, my daughter's name is India, like the country –

FEMALE REPRESENTATIVE NUMBER 43: That's real pretty-

OUR HEROINE: *(smelling a rat, but masking it with involuntary Midwestern politeness)* Thanks.

FEMALE REPRESENTATIVE NUMBER 43: Different. Can I get India's date of birth?

OUR HEROINE erroneously supplies her non-epileptic male child's date of birth, then scrambles to correct herself before her credibility is irreparably damaged in the eyes of her children's insurer.

FEMALE REPRESENTATIVE NUMBER 43: And if you'd just please verify your home address.

OUR HEROINE, teeth grinding, verifies her home address.

FEMALE REPRESENTATIVE NUMBER 43: Thank you for calling Sunspire. How may I assist you today?

OUR HEROINE: Okay, well, my daughter has this neurologist she sees regularly, and I just received this bill for seven hundred dollars—

FEMALE REPRESENTATIVE NUMBER 43: Can I get the physician's provider number?

OUR HEROINE: I don't have the number, but I know he participates with you guys. He's her regular neurolo—

FEMALE REPRESENTATIVE NUMBER 43: (*disproportionately merry*) Ha, ha, that's okay! I can find it using his name.

OUR HEROINE: Great. It's Head, Franklin Head; he used to be at Beth Elohim, now he's at -

FEMALE REPRESENTATIVE NUMBER 43: May I have the date the services were provided?

OUR HEROINE: (*Guiltily scans the top most statement in a collection of four, three of which have yet to be removed from their still-sealed envelopes*) Uh, last February?

FEMALE REPRESENTATIVE NUMBER 43: (*betraying no particular emotion*) All right, let's take a look at our records … hmm, okay, okay; I'm seeing that Monkeypants Pediatrics FAXed a preauthorization request for India to see Dr. Head on December 14, but that expired.

OUR HEROINE: But he's her regular guy. She's been seeing him since she was four!

FEMALE REPRESENTATIVE NUMBER 43: Unfortunately, in order for Sunspire to honor that claim, we would need for her primary provider, which in this case would be Monkeypants Pediatrics, to have FAXed through a new preauthorization request in advance of the appointment.

Simultaneously:
OUR HEROINE: Oh hmm, see, the thing is, though, I, I think they did. I mean, they're usually really on top of that sort of thing.
OUR HEROINE'S INTERIOR MONOLOGUE: Fuck, fuck, shit, shit, fuck me, she's right! I forgot about preauthorization! I probably forgot on purpose, because Dr. Monkeypants's receptionist gets so pissed when people leave it to the last minute instead of giving her a minimum of five days lead time! I hate talking on the phone! I hate myself!

FEMALE REPRESENTATIVE NUMBER 43: Okay, let's take a look. Yeah, hmm, all I'm seeing is that request from December.

OUR HEROINE: Oh… okay…uh…

FEMALE REPRESENTATIVE NUMBER 43: (*brightly*) The good thing is, once we do receive a request, it's good for three visits within one calendar year, so you don't have to call your pediatrician every time your daughter has got an appointment coming up.

OUR HEROINE: Yeah. Great. As far as this one goes, though, I'm still not sure what could've happened. I definitely remember calling and talking to the receptionist…do you think maybe she FAXed it to the wrong number?

FEMALE REPRESENTATIVE NUMBER 43: (*dryly*) I suppose that's possible.

OUR HEROINE: Is that the sort of thing that *could* happen, in your experience?

FEMALE REPRESENTATIVE NUMBER 43: I'd recommend calling your pediatrician. Maybe they have some sort of record they could FAX over.

OUR HEROINE: *(fatigued, two minutes shy of needing to leave to leave to pick the children up from school)* Okay. And then should I call you back?"

•　　•　　•

Scene Three
Enough time has elapsed that OUR HEROINE, the Conflict-Avoiding, Procrastination-Prone Artist Mother of the Epileptic Child, considers herself something of a hoary old vet, the type of person who conceivably could handle this sort of thing in her sleep.

We find her in a royal snit. The pharmacist she bakes cookies for every Christmas has made repeated attempts to refill the not-entirely-effective prescription drugs the epileptic child takes three times a day, but the stonewalling insurance company will not approve the transaction. According to the labels on the now-nearly-empty bottles, the epileptic child is entitled to four more refills before her mother must go against her nature and bug the neurologist for another six-month prescription. The greetings of the HEARTY AUTOMATED WHITE MALE and LESS-HEARTY, AUTOMATED, SPANISH-SPEAKING FEMALE are by now so familiar that OUR HEROINE barely registers them, reflexively stabbing the appropriate buttons on her telephone when asked. Then…

HEARTY AUTOMATED WHITE MALE: According to our records that policy has been cancelled.

OUR HEROINE: *(((silent scream)))*

•　　•　　•

Scene Four
Some fifteen seconds after Scene Three

Majorly freaking, OUR HEROINE immediately redials. Frantic in her desire to muscle past the prompts of HEARTY AUTOMATED WHITE MALE and LESS-HEARTY, AUTOMATED, SPANISH-SPEAKING FEMALE, she rasps "Representative!" every time she is asked to either make a selection or enter personal information. Finally…

FEMALE REPRESENTATIVE NUMBER 207: Hello, thank you for calling Sunspire Child Health Plus, my name is Debbie, may I-

OUR HEROINE, on the verge of having a seizure herself, verifies her identity, then gabbles incoherently about a policy she claims has been cancelled in error. She invokes epilepsy, as in serious we-ain't-playing epilepsy for which three different types of seizure suppressing medications must be taken three times a day. Apparently those medications have run out, and without insurance, she is incapable of procuring them in such quantities as will keep her daughter from suffering a mind-blowing, game-over seizure. OUR HEROINE leans heavily on her theatrical training, suspecting it to be the last, best option for someone like her, who, despite a fairly privileged upbringing and a college degree, has no idea how the system works! At least she has a fluent native speaker's command of English. Fuck fuck fuck fuck fuck!

FEMALE REPRESENTATIVE NUMBER 207: Mrs. Halliday, if it's all right with you, I'm just going to put you on hold for one moment while I check our records, see if we can figure out what's going on here.

OUR HEROINE: (*gratefully*) Yes, yes, please!

SOULLESS CAUCASIAN SINGERS: Do you know the way to San Jo—

FEMALE REPRESENTATIVE NUMBER 207: Okay, Mrs. Halliday, I pulled up your daughter's file, and unfortunately, I am seeing that that policy was cancelled due to non-payment on—

OUR HEROINE: *(sinking to her knees a la Willem Dafoe at the end of* Platoon... *Her college acting teacher would have no doubt objected to such untempered ham-handedness, but he is in Evanston, Illinois with a new crop of students, and she is alone in a New York City apartment, attempting to flounder her way out of the worst pickle of her life, a pickle that could have been avoided entirely by simple bill payment.)* But, but, but, oh my god. Oh god.

FEMALE REPRESENTATIVE NUMBER 207: *(stoic, but possibly seething with offense at hearing the Lord's name taken in vain)* I can send you an application if you'd like to reenroll—

OUR HEROINE: *(quickly)* Can we do that over the phone now?

FEMALE REPRESENTATIVE NUMBER 207: I'm afraid that's not possible, Mrs. Halliday.

OUR HEROINE: I can give you my Visa!

FEMALE REPRESENTATIVE NUMBER 207: I'm sorry, Mrs. Halliday, but our system is set up in such a way that even if I tried to reenroll you right now, the computer wouldn't let me. The best I can do is send you the application and have you return it to us in time for the beginning of the next billing cycle.

OUR HEROINE: *(assuming the prawn position)* Oh god. Oh god.

FEMALE REPRESENTATIVE NUMBER 207: Now, you should know that along with that application, we'll also be require a check for the overdue balance on the cancelled account, plus two months' payment on the new account, at whatever the current premium happens to be.

OUR HEROINE: But what are we supposed to do until then? She's got to have this medicine! Even with it, she has like five or six little seizures a day! She falls off the jungle gym at school! If she doesn't get it, she could—

FEMALE REPRESENTATIVE NUMBER 207: Mm, yes, that's why we recommend paying your statements as soon as you receive them.

Simultaneously:
OUR HEROINE: I know, I'm so sorry I fell behind, it's just I've had a lot on my plate recently and we were on vacation, and then, I, I, I...wait, do you think maybe if I came by with a check?
OUR HEROINE'S INTERIOR MONOLOGUE: Fuck you, lady! If my kid has a seizure and dies it's your fault! No! Take that back! Don't jinx yourself! Oh my god, I'm so fucked. I'm a danger to my own child. I'm a horrible, selfish moron! This nightmare is entirely my fault!

FEMALE REPRESENTATIVE NUMBER 207: We're in Blue Bonnet Shoals. That's right outside Albany.

OUR HEROINE: There's not some office in the city where I could—

FEMALE REPRESENTATIVE NUMBER 207: No.

Simultaneously:
OUR HEROINE'S INTERIOR MONOLOGUE: Fuck fuck shit fuck shit!!!
OUR HEROINE: Please! She's only got two pills left before she runs out!

Long, long Pause.

FEMALE REPRESENTATIVE NUMBER 207: Let me speak to my supervisor.

•   •   •

Scene Five
Three-and-a-half days and several dozen phone calls after Scene Four

HEARTY AUTOMATED WHITE MALE and LESS-HEARTY, AUTOMATED, SPANISH-SPEAKING FEMALE run through their customary spiels. OUR HEROINE, the Conflict-Avoiding, Procrastination-Prone Artist Mother of the Epileptic Child, clings hollow-eyed to something resembling a yogic breathing regimen, wincing as HEARTY AUTOMATED WHITE MALE reiterates that according to his records, this policy has been cancelled.

FEMALE REPRESENTATIVE NUMBER 214: Thank you for calling Sunspire. My name is Cheryl Case. May—

OUR HEROINE: I'm calling about my daughter. Her account was cancelled because I screwed up the bill, but I spoke with Debbie on Thursday and she spoke with Mr. Toms and he said as long as I could get a check to you by today, the policy could be reinstated, which is really critical because she takes all this seizure medication for epilepsy. I was able to get the pharmacist to sell me a few pills to get us through the weekend, but –

FEMALE REPRESENTATIVE NUMBER 214 *interrupts to have OUR HEROINE verify her identity. Dutifully supplied. The account remains cancelled. Oh god. Oh no. Oh fuckfuckfuckfuck no!!!!*

OUR HEROINE: *(wild-eyed, frothing)* But, but, I sent the check on Thursday, right after I got off the phone with Debbie!

FEMALE REPRESENTATIVE NUMBER 214: You sent it to the address in Blue Bonnet Shoals, not the PO Box on the bill?

OUR HEROINE: Yes! Yes!!!

FEMALE REPRESENTATIVE NUMBER 214: Okay, do you have the Fed Ex tracking number?

OUR HEROINE: *(bowels freezing with regret)* I didn't send it Fed Ex.

FEMALE REPRESENTATIVE NUMBER 214: According to Debbie's notes, you were told to Fed Ex a check for the full amount for overnight delivery, with the understanding that we needed to receive that check by today in order to reinstate the account?

OUR HEROINE: *(barely audible)* I know but the lady at the UPS store said that since we're both in New York, and the post office was just a block away, Priority Mail would be just as good.

FEMALE REPRESENTATIVE NUMBER 214: *(Pause.)* Let me get this straight. You were at a place where you could send it via Fed Ex, and then you decided to go to the post office instead?

OUR HEROINE: I know.

FEMALE REPRESENTATIVE NUMBER 214: So, you sent it via USPS, Priority Overnight?

OUR HEROINE: *(ashen)* No, just regular Priority.

FEMALE REPRESENTATIVE NUMBER 214: Even though you understood that that check absolutely, no exceptions, had to be in our hands by Friday.

OUR HEROINE: *(Childlike in her wretchedness)* She said it would be just as fast.

FEMALE REPRESENTATIVE NUMBER 214: Did you at least send it certified or request delivery confirmation?

OUR HEROINE: No, I… I used the automated machine in the lobby.

FEMALE REPRESENTATIVE NUMBER 214: *(under her breath)* Incredible.

OUR HEROINE: *(sadly)* Believe me, I'm kicking myself for not sending it Fed Ex. I guess I was thinking it would be a good thing to save twenty bucks. Stupid.

Defeated, OUR HEROINE stares at the cheap, boob-shaped overhead fixture in her cramped, $1,400/month living room, agonized that she is so immature as to have lapses during which her responsibility for her child's health seems less of a priority than checking her email, or pursuing some half-baked artsy whim. Would that the precious creature had never been stricken, that health was a thing that could be taken blissfully for granted until some day in the extremely far distant future when OUR HEROINE, herself, is painlessly and poignantly expiring, surrounded by loving family members and high-thread count linens.

FEMALE REPRESENTATIVE NUMBER 214: You do understand that a huge exception was being made in your case?

OUR HEROINE: *(Lord Jesus, have pity on this miserable sinner…she knows not what she does…)* I know. It's my fault that I screwed it up.

FEMALE REPRESENTATIVE NUMBER 214: *(sighs, murderously sick of dealing with incompetents such as this hippie dippy ding dong.)* All right. What did the envelope you mailed it in look like?

OUR HEROINE: *(arm hair prickling, alert)* What?

FEMALE REPRESENTATIVE NUMBER 214: There's a *chance* it might have been delivered this morning, but we get thousands of pieces of mail every day. Maybe it's sitting in a bin in the mailroom.

OUR HEROINE: It was one of those red, white and blue Flat Rate envelopes.

FEMALE REPRESENTATIVE NUMBER 214: Great. I hope you don't have anywhere to be because this might take a while.

OUR HEROINE: I can hold!

FEMALE REPRESENTATIVE NUMBER 214: There's no guarantee that it's there.

OUR HEROINE: *(Experiencing the adrenalin rush of a woman wrenching the roof off a car to free her infant from a flaming wreck)* No, no, I know! Take all the time you need!

FEMALE REPRESENTATIVE NUMBER 214: *(no love in her voice)* All right. Please hold.

(An interval of nearly twenty minutes. Cue string heavy instrumentals of various soft rock hits. OUR HEROINE psyches herself up. She must be like the mother puma, ready to hop a Greyhound bus four hours north to Albany in order to sort through the insurance company's mail for them! She hopes security clearance will not be a problem. She hopes another mother will volunteer to pick up her children from school for her, because no way will she be back in time. She cringes to imagine how much a cab to Blue Bonnet Shoals will run her, but whatever the cost, she has lost the privilege to bitch about it. Her heartbeat rivals that of a hummingbird's.)

At last:
FEMALE REPRESENTATIVE NUMBER 214: *(grudgingly)* Well, you're in luck. We found it in one of the last bins we looked in.

(Cue offstage celestial choir)

OUR HEROINE: OH MY GOD!!! Thank you!!!!

FEMALE REPRESENTATIVE NUMBER 214: You do understand that this was a one-time thing. If you fail to pay on time again, we won't be able to—

OUR HEROINE: *(determined to prove that she will do better, that she will never ever fuck up again, that from here on out all will be smooth sailing and conscious, timely effort, the margin for human error all used up, and thus, permanently eliminated.)* I understand! It was my one get out of jail free card and after that no more. Thank you! And please, tell Debbie and Mr. Toms thank you from me too!

FEMALE REPRESENTATIVE NUMBER 214: I'll reinstate your daughter's account as of today. It may take a few hours to go through.

OUR HEROINE (*Scheming to mail cookies to the address in Blue Bonnet Shoals. For one reason and another, she will not get around to actually doing so for another week and a half, and will worry that they will arrive stale, but she sort of knows the recipients have cemented their opinion of her, and probably wouldn't be too grateful even if the unsolicited treat had been Fed-Exed straight out of the oven*) Oh my god, I can't thank you enough!

FEMALE REPRESENTATIVE NUMBER 214 disconnects without thanking OUR HEROINE for calling Sunspire.

OUR HEROINE collapses on the carpet and remains there until shortly before she is due to pick up her children from school. For once, she does not feel guilty about failing to use her child-free time in pursuit of some negligible artistic goal.

• • •

DISCUSSION GUIDE:

How does the author's tendency to avoid conflict, procrastinate, and preoccupy herself with artistic goals of no discernible impact influence her ongoing negotiations with her children's insurance provider?

Why might someone in the author's position not sign up for automatic bill pay?

Why might the children's father balk at stripping the author of all duties relating to the children's health insurance?

How many times in the last year have you heard the word "seizure" used in a humorous, non-epileptic context?

Did you know Mark Twain had an epileptic child who suffered a fatal seizure on Christmas Day?

Did you know that the title character in *Carrie* was partially based on an epileptic girl Stephen King knew in high school, who died of a massive seizure in her 20s?

The author has another character allude to her as a "hippie ding dong," albeit nonverbally. Is this an apt description? If so, why do you think she is relying three different types of prescription medication to semi-control her child's seizures, as opposed to herbs, crystals, and creative visualization?

How does the author's nationality influence or define her experience?

How might these scenes have played out prior to the advent of the automated-phone-system?

Why are all the female representatives female?

Might the author's attitude be a chronic reflection of the fact that she doesn't like to talk on the phone?

Do you think the author has "learned her lesson" by the end of this piece?

Why would the original publisher wait until the last minute to request that the author cut scene five from the finished piece, so as not to lose the reader's sympathy?

Why might the author, despite her ingrained Midwestern desire to be liked by all, refuse?

Would the author seem more sympathetic had she majored in business administration or something less frivolous than an archaic art form that rarely translates to a living wage?

What if the author's child had leukemia or cystic fibrosis? What about autism, asthma, or a severe peanut allergy?

What will happen when the author's child is no longer eligible for 'Sunspire Child Health Plus'? Is that 18 or 19? It's not like a new insurer could deny her coverage based on a pre-existing condition, or could they? Do we trust the author to begin researching the answers to this question in a timely manner?

Wouldn't it be totally awesome if the author's child's epilepsy spontaneously cured itself?

Originally published in *My Baby Rides the Short Bus.*

MAKING IT HOME TO YOURSELF

Juniper Tree

By the time I was 24 years old, I already had a lot of health problems. I found the amount of care I need affects my ability to participate fully in this world. However, I am healing and learning to see the positive aspects of taking care of myself. I am starting to ally myself with my weaknesses and appreciate myself for all that I have been through and am capable of doing in this lifetime.

I struggle with Adrenal Fatigue, hypoglycemia, Polycystic Ovarian Syndrome (PCOS), an inguinal hernia in my right groin, and digestion issues. I also have multiple food allergies and the list is growing. I was raised eating the Standard American Diet until I was 19 years old when I cut out gluten, dairy, soy, sugar, caffeine, and processed foods.

Understanding Adrenal Fatigue and what causes it has been important to my healing. This condition occurs when one's adrenal glands cannot adequately meet the demands of physical, emotional, psychological, spiritual, or environmental stress. Over-stimulation of one's adrenals can be caused by a very intense single stress or by chronic or repeated stresses that have a cumulative effect.

I was diagnosed at 15 years old due to a stressful home environment as a child. My parents argued a lot, my mother had a heart attack when I was 10; my brother struggled with mental health issues since I was little, I did not have any positive adult role models, and I endured a lot of verbal abuse from people who were supposed to love me.

Adrenal Fatigue means the body thinks it needs to be in a constant fight or flight response. Everything I do on a daily basis is part of this feedback loop. Someone unexpectedly comes into the house and with my nervous system on edge, I am ready to defend or run. The dog barks at the mailman who comes every single day at the same time and I jump, usually followed by a release of energy in the form of a cuss word. My mouth is dry, I am always thirsty, and I have to pee constantly. Sometimes after sitting for a long time, I feel dizzy upon standing. I find myself completely surrendering to anxiety, worry, and compulsive thinking habits. I feel nervous and insecure in my body and not all "here."

My heart rate is usually fast and when I am nervous I sweat profusely. I feel brain fog and have a scattered yet obsessive memory. My brain wants to make sure that I am completely safe. It protects me so that I will not forget anything I need, making sure I have not lost any of my possessions through the transitions of life. At various points in my life my rights were taken away without my consent. Adrenal Fatigue is a coping mechanism my body has developed for survival.

One of my most residual traumas was mandatory schooling at a Catholic middle/high school. It was here that my self-esteem, my ability to speak up for myself, and my ability to share my opinions was severely injured. I pretended that I could not hear anything the jerks said to me or about me. I refused to grace them with the presence of my lovely voice. I felt like no one liked me and I had no friends. My anxiety was through the roof. I spent every hour of every waking day pouring myself endlessly into my notebook; my haven, my safe zone, the place where I could be completely honest and full of integrity.

I do not feel comfortable shining in this world due to the messages I received while growing up. I fear that if I shine, no one will like me, telling me everything I was told for years; that I am a fake, a tease, that I am not good enough, and wishy-washy. I fear it will all be confirmed by current notions of my character. I know this is simply not true, yet it remains difficult to fully reject these doubts.

We need to grow in accepting our sexuality, in feeling attractive in our bodies, in accepting who we are attracted to and why. We need to accept genuine love from ourselves and others who truly care. We need to grow in our gender identities and expression of who we are through the way we dress and speak. It is important to gain more confidence in sharing political opinions, visions for our lives, and visions for community building and sustainable living. We need to accept the beauty of our bodies as well as tell others they are beautiful. We need to share our beautiful words, art, and songs with the world. We need to learn to show up in our bodies so that others can see us for who we truly are. And I need to stop pretending and apologizing for myself.

I am growing in these areas and am grateful to be working on myself at this time in my life. My health problems have improved thanks to the supportive healing community I have found in Yellow Springs, Ohio. I spend two nights a month in circle with women celebrating the New and

Full moons, singing, dancing and sharing deeply. I have found a lot of healing in drum circles, and in a practice called Authentic Movement. I received monetary support from a local organization that has allowed me to see an acupuncturist and I barter with a chiropractor. I am getting the care, support, and love I need. I am growing and changing more than I ever could have imagined.

I came to Yellow Springs in 2006 to attend Antioch College where I was heavily influenced by anarchist ideas and movements. I had my own perspective from my experiences of authority, religion, and power dynamics within my family that laid the groundwork for my education. Over time I found that identifying as an anarchist has been healing because it fosters my belief in the genuine capacity for all of human kind to cooperate and create healthy societies. It is empowering to embrace an ideology and lifestyle that brings meaning and commitment to my life. Embracing anarchism can be a road to discovering our true selves and our true potential.

There is an interview with anarchist David Graeber where he defines anarchism as "the commitment to the idea that it would be possible to have a society based on principles of self-organization, voluntary association, and mutual aid." To relate to anarchism in this manner gives me hope that comes from each of us and spreads to all of our relationships with family, friends, lovers, and community members.

It energizes me to be a part of activism. It is my outlet for bringing my ideals into the world, yet I find myself unsure of where it fits into my life. I make just enough money to buy supplements and healthy food and most of my energy is directed toward taking care of myself. In my experience it has been difficult to participate in movements with my food restrictions and physical and emotional health limitations. I don't feel that I am of assistance to resistance movements unless I have a solid foundation on which I thrive. I see no other way to be an activist than to value my need to heal. I do not have to be an isolated person meeting her own needs and ignoring everyone else.

I see my health education as my activism and realizing that I can use my journey of gathering knowledge and resources to teach others. An integral part of my healing process has been settling into my body and building a safe life. A definition of safety I found is, "To feel free to be oneself, to feel that your emotional and physical well being are not in any jeopardy from outside forces." I want to be a part of a holistic health community where we all care for one another, relearning, remembering our roots and severing those ties to the lies we were taught.

A lot of people do not have access to the support I have found, nor do they have the time or resources to focus on their deep needs. I see this issue through a class, race, and gender lens. Billions of people are grieving the loss of their homelands, families, and stolen futures. My message is that we are worth the time and energy of taking care of ourselves. Infrastructure needs to be created for these spaces and ideas to take root in people of all backgrounds and socioeconomic statuses.

The journey of individuation is lonely but the deepest part within my soul is telling me this is worthwhile work. The original meaning of the word courage was *"To speak one's mind by telling all of one's heart."* This is what I hope to leave this planet knowing I have done. When I feel lost in other's expectations of me, I consult my moral compass, the place where True North and True Self never waiver. I listen to the deep stirrings within myself, heed the wisdom of my body's symptoms, and give myself what I truly need in the moment. Healing, I have decided, is my path and my true challenge now is to stick to it.

if you eat well
get physical
exercise
dont smoke
tobacco
drink alcohol
moderately
you will win

SUBSCRIBE TO EVERYTHING WE PUBLISH!

Do you love what Microcosm publishes?

Do you want us to publish more great stuff?

Would you like to receive each new title as it's published?

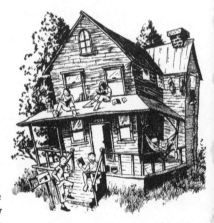

Subscribe as a BFF to our new titles and we'll mail them all to you as they are released!

$10-30/mo, pay what you can afford. Include your t-shirt size and month/date of birthday for a possible surprise! Subscription begins the month after it is purchased.

microcosmpublishing.com/bff